EROTIC MASSAGE

The Tantric Touch of Love

Kenneth Ray Stubbs, Ph.D.

with
Louise-Andrée Saulnier

Illustrated
by
Kyle Spencer

Jeremy P. Tarcher/Putnam
a member of
Penguin Putnam Inc.
New York

Most Tarcher/Putnam books are available at special quantity discounts for bulk purchase for sales promotions, premiums, fund-raising, and educational needs. Special books or book excerpts also can be created to fit specific needs. For details, write Putnam Special Markets, 375 Hudson Street, New York, NY 10014.

A Word of Caution

The purpose of this book is to educate. It is not intended to give medical or psychological therapy. Whenever there is concern about physical or emotional illness, a qualified professional should be consulted.

The authors, illustrators, and the publisher shall have neither liability nor responsibility to any person or entity with respect to any loss, damage, injury, or ailment caused or alleged to be caused directly or indirectly by the information or lack of information in this book.

Jeremy P. Tarcher/Putnam
a member of
Penguin Putnam Inc.
375 Hudson Street
New York, NY 10014
www.penguinputnam.com

First Jeremy P. Tarcher edition 1998
Originally published by Secret Garden, Larkspur, California
Copyright © 1989, 1993 by Kenneth Ray Stubbs, Ph.D.

Illustrations by Kyle Spencer
Based on Photography by Ellen Gunther
Chapter Heading Artwork by Richard Stodart

Library of Congress Cataloging-in-Publication Data

Stubbs, Kenneth Ray.
    Erotic massage : the tantric touch of love / Kenneth Ray Stubbs.
        p.   cm.
    Rev. ed. of: Tantric massage, an illustrated manual for meditative sexuality. New York (?) ; Secret Garden, 1993.
    ISBN 0-87477-962-6 (alk. paper)
    1. Sex instruction.   2. Massage.   I. Title.
HQ31.S97   1999   98-33371 CIP
613.9'6—dc21

Printed in the United States of America
                17 18 19 20

This book is printed on acid-free paper. ∞

Acceptance
       is a central teaching
       in tantric traditions
Embracing the whole,
       we transcend
          the world of duality

Today in the West
       tantra
          has often come to mean
      sacred sex, spiritual sexuality, sexual spirituality
It is in this context
       that I use
tantric massage:
       touching
          the sexual and spiritual dimensions
             within each of us
          —with full acceptance
          —embracing an apparent duality

Dedicated to

Suzanne Myers
and
Paul Fleming

Your gifts are remembered.

CONTENTS

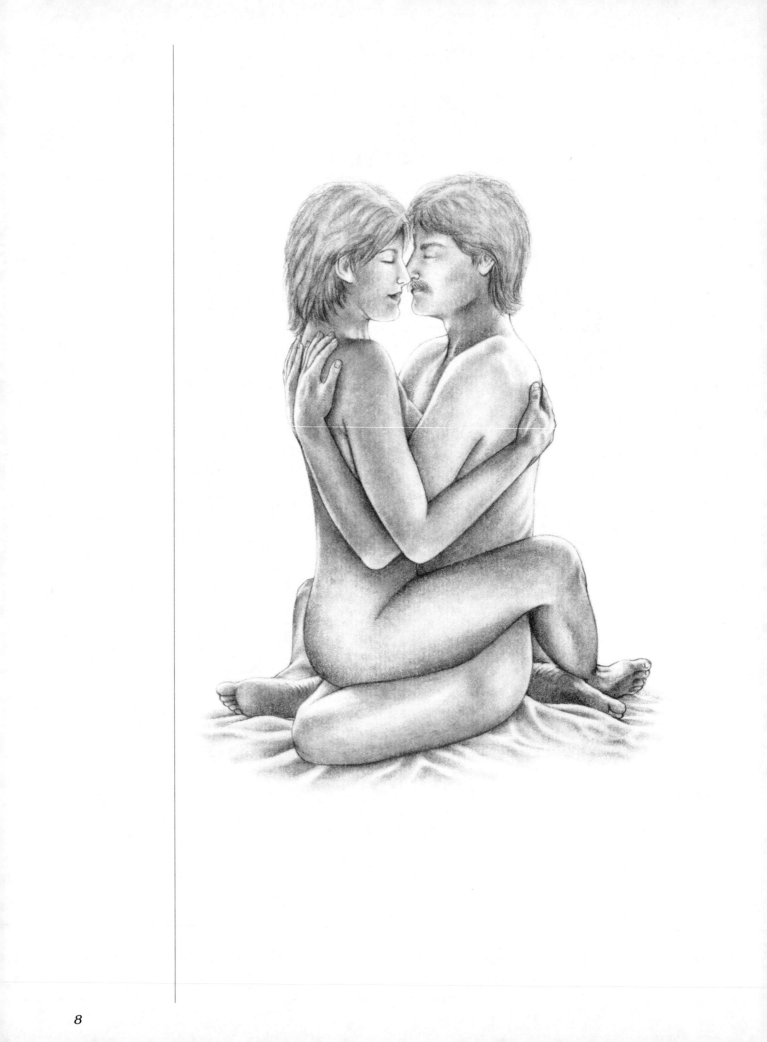

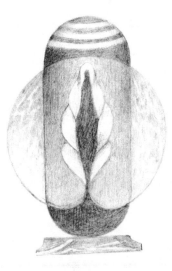

INVITATION

This is a language
without words

This is a time
outside of time

This is a song
that sings
a celebration

This is the meditation of massage

INTRODUCTION

Massage
      is a dance of energy

Massage
      is a dance of love

This is a love book especially for lovers
      Your boyfriend, your girlfriend
      your wife
      your husband
      your significant other, your lover, your mate
         the label is not important
      the feeling is

You may be friends
      exploring becoming lovers

You may be lovers
      exploring becoming friends

What is most important
         is that
what you do
      is
consensual

Massage simply stated
        simply is
    patterned touch
We might say
    a caress
    is unpatterned touch
Which you choose to give
    or to receive
    depends on the mood
Be open to either
    Both heal
    Both nurture
    Both excite

During the massage
    either or both of you
        might feel erotic
    You might fall asleep
    You might burst out in laughter
        or in tears

You might or might not
    have sex before
        during
        or after
    However, should sex or orgasm become
        the goal,
    you might miss
    many other pleasures

Allow each moment
        each feeling
    to unfold
    itself
This is the meditation

Massage
      is an art
            when you
      express yourself
            with sensitivity
            with awareness

Let your touch
discover
      without demands
      without expectations

At first
      the techniques
      will be
      techniques,
            like learning
            to ride a bicycle
After a while
      the awkward will become
      familiar

Your touch
      will come
      to nourish
the body
the mind
      and
the spirit

You will also find
      your beloved's body
            — in stillness —
      pleasuring your hands
Let your fingertips
      taste
            the curve
            the rough, the smooth
            the firm
            the soft

Let yourself feel

WHAT YOU NEED

A willing recipient

A quiet place

A warm place
       or if it is tropical,
       gentle breezes

Oil, perhaps a lotion
       — on membranous tissue,
         a water-based lubricant
         may be healthier

A towel

A padded table
       a bed or padded floor
       or a large towel
         on the beach

Gentle music, if you wish

Perhaps
       feathers
       a silk scarf

MEDITATIVE MASSAGE
GUIDELINES

Three basic ones:

First and foremost
    be present
Letting go of expectations
    of the future
        and
    comparisons with the past,
Be
    Here
Be

    Now

Secondly
    maintain full-hand contact
        whenever possible
    Allow your palms
        fingers
        and thumbs
    to outline the contours

Thirdly
    maintain a continuous flow
Movements blend together,
    each one
    enhancing the preceding one
    and preparing the next

More important
> than the techniques
>> is
> your own personal expression

More important than
> your own personal expression
>> is
> the recipient's wishes

More important than
> the recipient's wishes
>> is
> your never forcing yourself

Yet
> be open to discovering
> new horizons

It's a delicate dance

REMINDERS

If the sensation
     feels good to the recipient,
     you are doing it correctly,
          regardless
          of theory or written instructions

Vary
     the pressure
     the tempo
     the rhythm
Repeating a stroke in the exact same way each time
     becomes boring very quickly
     to both the recipient and the giver

If there are two of them,
     massage both

Glide on and off
     To begin a touch,
          rather than plopping on
     glide on with a slow descent
          in the direction
          that your hands will be moving
     In coming off
          continue the movement in a gradual ascent

Generally, minimize landings and takeoffs

When in doubt
     lighter pressure might be better
The recipient's preference, however,
     is the best guide
     Ask occasionally, if you are uncertain

Minimize the talking
An important exception:
      when the recipient needs
      to communicate deep feelings

Become centered
      Tuning into and slowing your breath
         you can quieten yourself

Being centered
      you will experience more deeply
      your own pleasure

The following strokes assume
      the massage is on a table
Except for some of the long strokes
      most of the instructions can be adapted
      to floor or bed massages

Follow the presented sequence
      or create a sequence
      more suitable for your situation

Massage the whole body
      or only one section

HEALTH

Discussing health concerns
     is essential
     in establishing trust
     in a relationship,
          whether it be for an evening
          or a lifetime

If a partner has a cold or flu,
     the other partner can choose
     to be close
     or not

If there is an infectious condition on the skin,
     forgo contact with that area
     Perhaps keep it clothed

If there is a concern
     about viral conditions
     communicable through bodily fluids,
          share your feelings with your partner
     Read this book's appendix,
          Eroticizing Safer-Sex
     Consult agencies promoting healthy sex
          and read literature
          which can assist you in choosing for yourself
          what is best
          in your sensual and sexual expressions

Ask if there are any tender places
Be especially gentle there
     or exclude
If an injury is severe
     or if there are circulation problems,
     first consult a health professional

The debates continue
> regarding the relative healthiness
> of vegetable oil
>> mineral oil
>> and water-based lubricants
> for massage on or in the body
Many commercial preparations contain
> preservatives, artificial colors
>> and other chemical additives
> Some people are allergic
>> to added fragrances
You may have to experiment first

Regarding conception
> please make parenthood planned

Now you are ready
> to make the final preparations
> for your special gift

PREPARATIONS

Where?

Anywhere
    as long as distractions
    and interruptions
        are minimized

Inside or outside is fine
    When outside,
        take precautions
        for insects and excessive sun
    When inside,
        unplug the phone
    Arrange for everyone else
        including children
    not to interrupt

It is very important
    to maintain a warm temperature
    If necessary, use a portable heater
        or cover the areas of the body
        you are not massaging at the moment

When?

Explore the energies of
    a full moon, a new moon
    an equinox, a solstice

Celebrate a birthday
    an anniversary
    Give a holiday-season present
        handmade

After intense work
    during a stressful period

Sometimes you can be spontaneous
  but setting aside a specific day or evening
    is more likely
    to ensure it happening

To give massage to a pregnant partner,
    is a gift not forgotten
  In the later stages
    she may be unable to lie on her front or back
  Perhaps forego some strokes or positions
    but not the touch

With What?

Basically all you need is oil
  fragranced ones entice the mind
    but may sting the skin
    especially membranous tissue
Some prefer vegetable oils
  (unfragranced coconut oil is a good choice)
  others prefer mineral oils
    Visit your local lotions-and-potions store,
      try a health food store
On membranous tissues, such as the female genitals,
  some consider water-based lubricants
  to be healthier
    Purchase them at a pharmacy
    perhaps at a sensuous boutique
You can apply the oil or lubricant to your hands
  either from a plastic squeeze bottle
  a bottle with a push pump
  or a bowl

Massage tables are great for your back
  and sturdy tabletops
    padded with foam or blankets are fine
  Otherwise, a padded floor
    a bed
    or the ground covered with cloth
    is quite suitable

If you select a large bed
  have the recipient's head
    at a corner of the foot of the bed
    while his/her feet are pointing toward
    the opposite corner at the head of the bed
  This will give you better access
    to both the right and left sides

For the covering cloth
  select a sheet or material
  that is OK to be oiled
    Some fabrics are difficult to clean
    and the oily smell may not wash out

Gather a large towel or two

When lying on the front side
       the recipient may need a covered foam pad
          or a couple of rolled towels
       placed under the front of the ankles

When lying on the back
       if there is strain in the lower back
       place the same pad underneath the knees

If you anticipate using feathers
          or other tactile stimulators
       have them close at hand

Perhaps select some music
       without dominating rhythms
       without words — usually

Use candlelight or colored lights
       incense
       flowers
       interior design of the room
          or whatever creates a special ambience
       However
       you do not have to create a temple every time
Sometimes
       all that is necessary
          is
       to close the door

Everything ready?

Oil

    phone unplugged
    temperature warm enough
    watches, jewelry, clothing removed
    recipient's contact lenses taken out (if necessary)
    your fingernails smoothed
    your hands cleaned and warmed?

Ask if any strokes
    on any particular places
    would be particularly pleasing

Ask for other possible relevancies
    such as preferences for no oil in the hair
    or time limitations

Once your beloved
      is ready to begin
    give the invitation
      to take a few fuller breaths
        and
      to close his/her eyes

Allowing
      your hands
      to move intuitively
    you can open doors
      to inner peace
      to pleasure
      to joy
    both your beloved's
      and
    yours

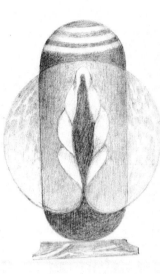

THE
MASSAGE
THE
MEDITATION

BEGINNING

Lover's Position:	Lying front down with arms by side.
Your Position:	Initially at your lover's left side.

1.
Laying On Of
Hands
1. A

1. Laying On Of Hands

A.
Center yourself.
Tune into your breathing.

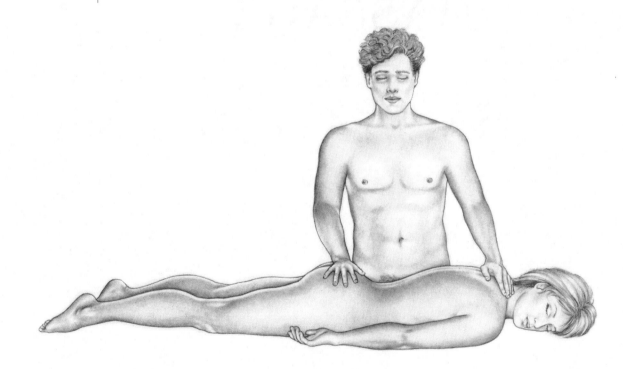

1. B

B.
Rest your left palm on the upper back,
your right palm on the sacrum.

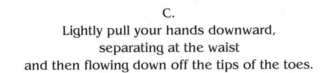

Laying On Of
Hands

C.
Lightly pull your hands downward,
separating at the waist
and then flowing down off the tips of the toes.

If you have feathers
or other sensuous materials,
stroke your lover
— all over —
now
before you apply any oil.

1. C

2. Spreading Oil

A.
Warm oil in your hands.
(Be careful not to let drops fall on your partner.)

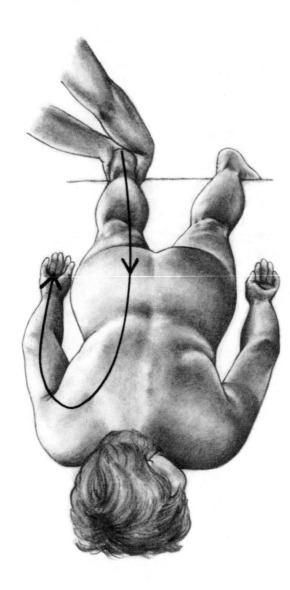

B.
Spread the oil by sliding your hands
up the back side:
starting at the feet, pull up the legs, the torso,
all the way off the fingertips.

~

Repeat the same sequence on the other side.
(It is easier if you first move to the other side.)

This is not the only oil application.
Generally, you add more oil
in the initial stroke of each section.

BACK

Your Position: Initially at your lover's head and facing his/her feet.

3. Connecting Stroke

3.
Connecting
Stroke

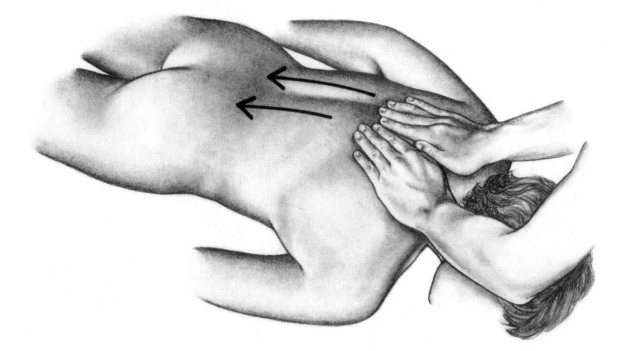

A.
Slide your parallel palms down the back
to the buttocks.

3. A

Connecting
Stroke

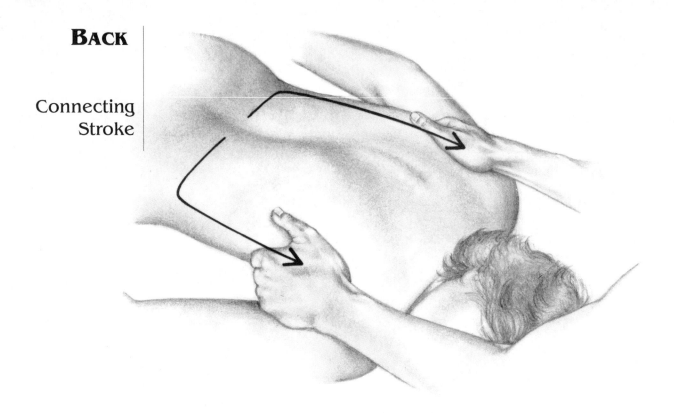

3. B

B.
Slide your palms outward to the sides of the waist
and then up the sides to the shoulders.

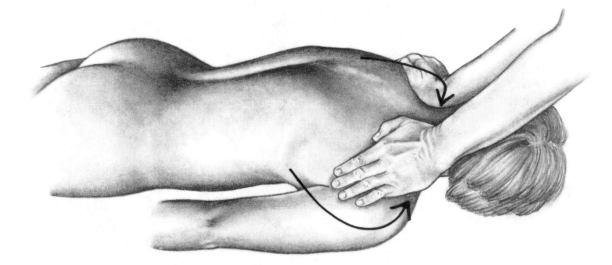

3. C

C.
On the shoulders, pivot your hands outward.

Connecting Stroke

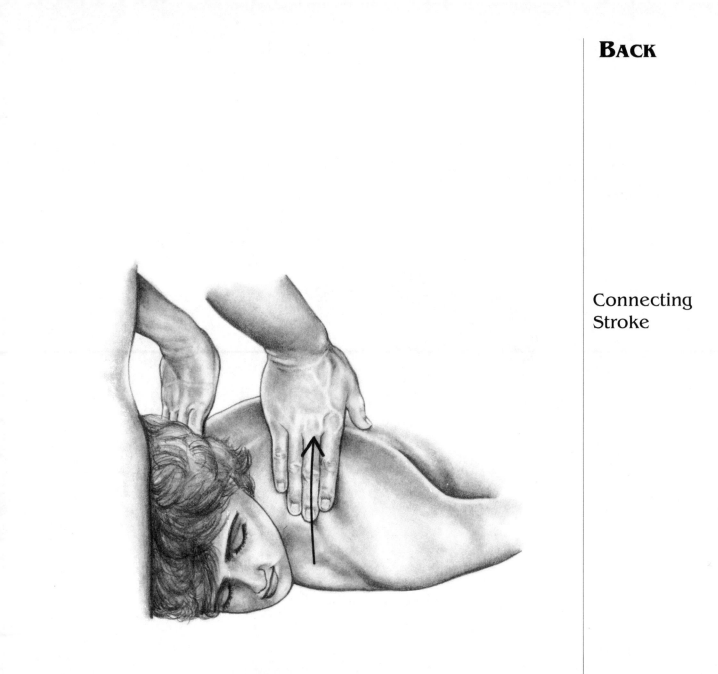

D.
Slide upwards across the shoulder muscles
(not the throat).

~

Repeat this whole stroke (A-D) several times.

3. D

4. Prayer Stroke

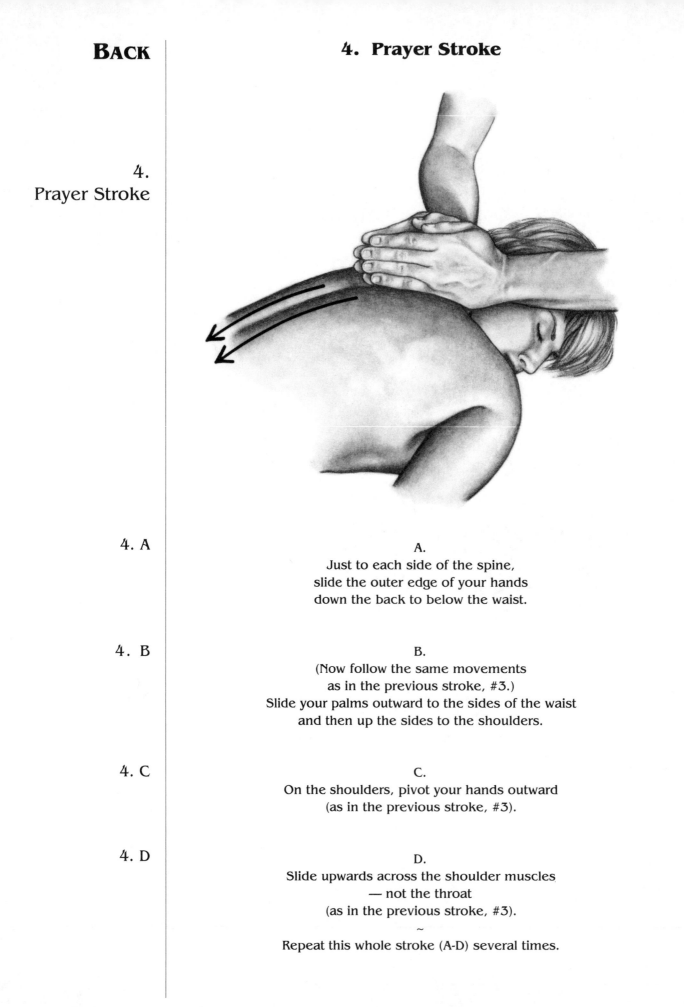

4.
Prayer Stroke

4. A

A.
Just to each side of the spine,
slide the outer edge of your hands
down the back to below the waist.

4. B

B.
(Now follow the same movements
as in the previous stroke, #3.)
Slide your palms outward to the sides of the waist
and then up the sides to the shoulders.

4. C

C.
On the shoulders, pivot your hands outward
(as in the previous stroke, #3).

4. D

D.
Slide upwards across the shoulder muscles
— not the throat
(as in the previous stroke, #3).

~

Repeat this whole stroke (A-D) several times.

5. Shoulder Strokes

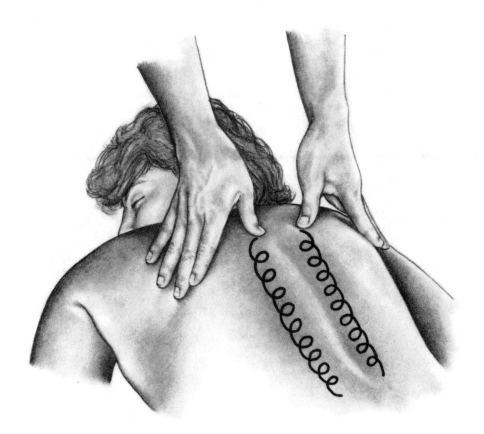

A.
Just to each side of the spine,
make circles with the flat parts of your thumbs.
Here the thumbs mirror each other:
down together,
outward from spine together,
etc.

Focus the pressure
in the direction toward his/her feet.
Let your fingers remain in contact with your partner.

This series of circles gradually comes UP the back.

**Shoulder
Strokes**

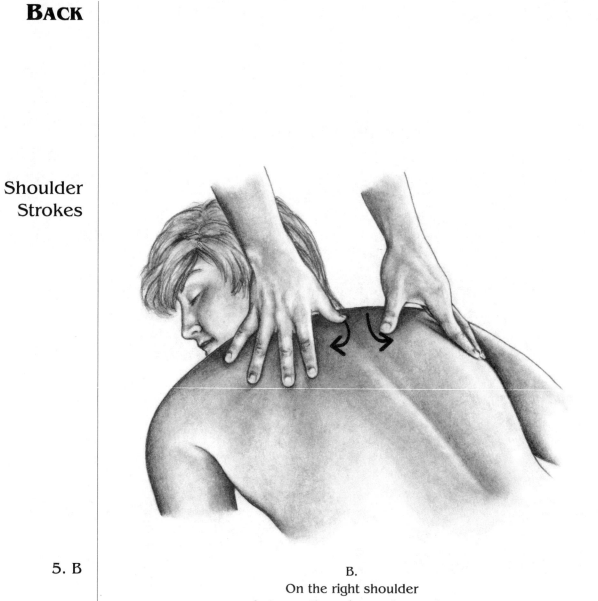

5. B

B.
On the right shoulder
between the spine and scapula,
make circles with your thumbs
— this time alternating your hands
one after the other.

Focus on the area near the neck.

Shoulder Strokes

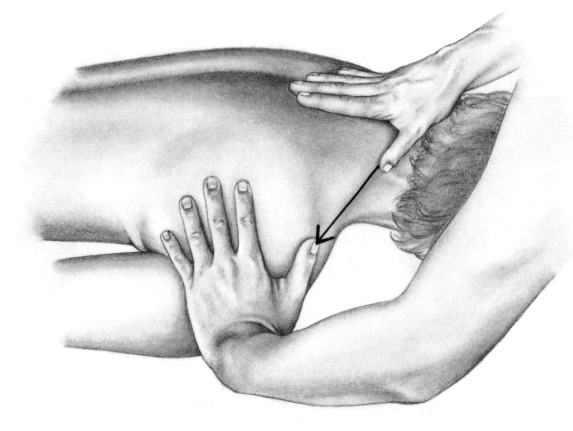

C.
On the groove
between the right scapula and clavicle,
slide your thumbs outward toward the shoulder tip
— alternating one hand after the other.

5. C

D.
Now apply Parts B and C on the left shoulder.

5. D

6.
Fingers' Pull

6. Fingers' Pull

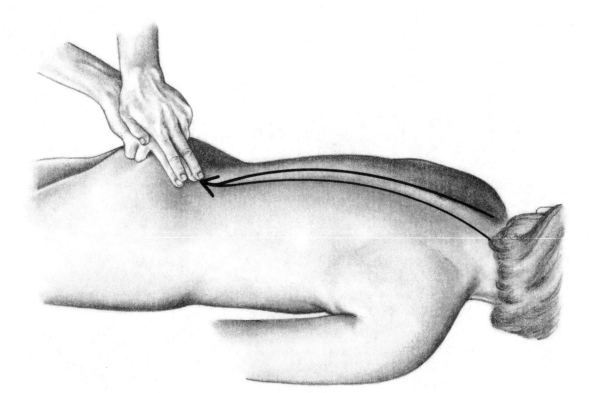

With a finger pad
on each side of the spine at the neck,
pull downward toward the buttocks.
Use a firm pressure.
(You can have even more pressure
by putting the fingers of your other hand
on top of the first.)

~

Repeat this whole stroke several times.

7. Side Pulling

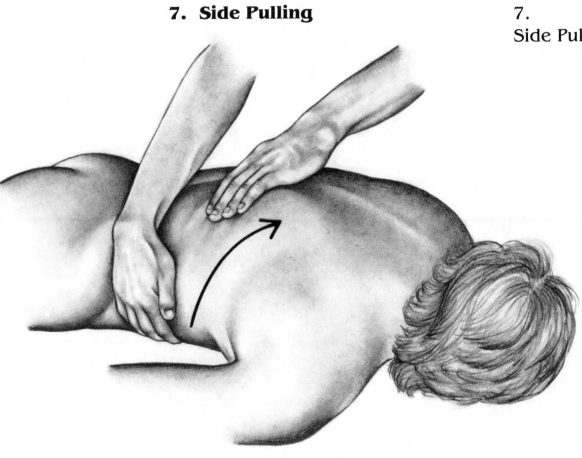

A.
Alternating your hands on one side,
slide them in a pulling manner
across the side of the torso
toward the spine.

(This series includes the area from the hips
to near the underarms.)

B.
Move to the other side,
and apply the pulling movements
to the opposite side.

BACK OF LEGS

Instructions: Written as applied to the right leg.
Your Position: Initially, to the right of the right foot.

8.
Connecting
Stroke

8. Connecting Stroke

8. A

A.
With your right hand in front,
slide your hands up the back of the leg.

(For both hands, the little-finger-side leads;
the thumbs are beside their index fingers.)

Connecting
Stroke

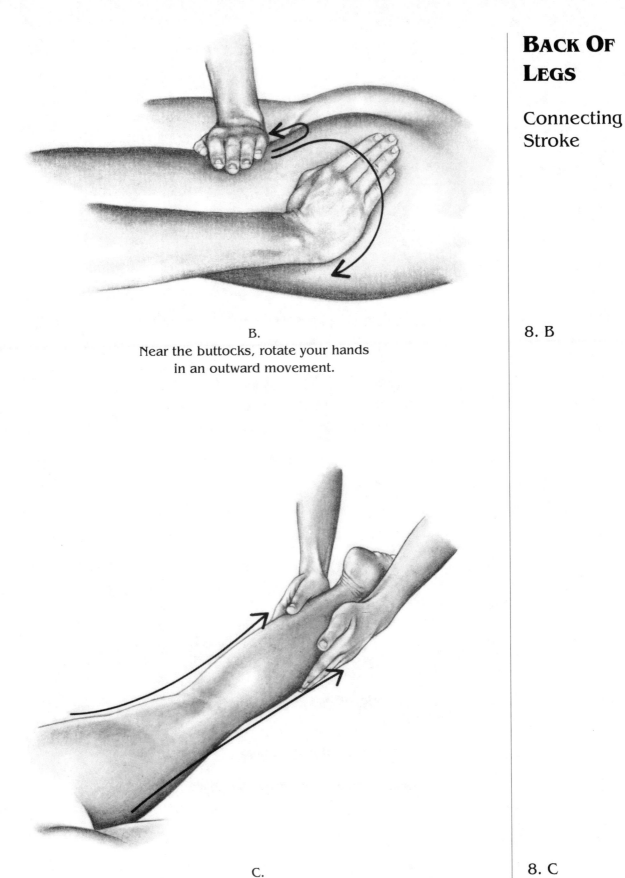

B.
Near the buttocks, rotate your hands
in an outward movement.

8. B

C.
Slide (in a pulling manner)
down the inner and outer sides of the leg.

~

Repeat this whole stroke (A-C) several times.

8. C

9.
Kneading

9. Kneading

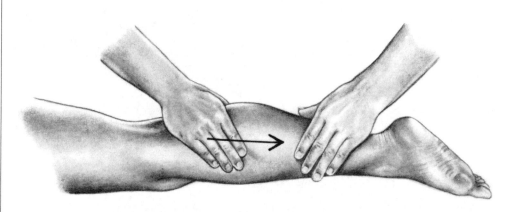

A. First focusing on one hand, gently squeeze
with your thumb opposite your fingers.
While squeezing, slide a few inches in the direction of your other hand.
Next release your squeeze.

B. Then follow the same pattern with the other hand.

Gradually knead the entire calf, thigh, and buttocks.

10. Thumb Slide

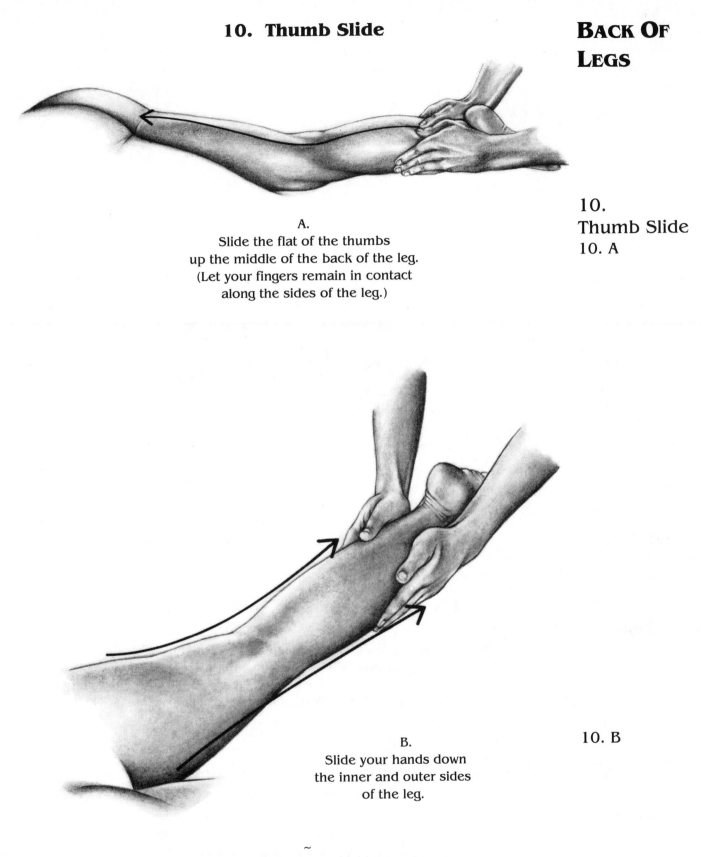

A.
Slide the flat of the thumbs
up the middle of the back of the leg.
(Let your fingers remain in contact
along the sides of the leg.)

B.
Slide your hands down
the inner and outer sides
of the leg.

10. B

~
Repeat this whole stroke (A-B) several times.

BACK OF LEGS

11.
V Stroke

11. A

11. B

12.
Repeat #8

13.
Feather Stroke

14.
Same
Sequence on
Left Leg

11. V Stroke

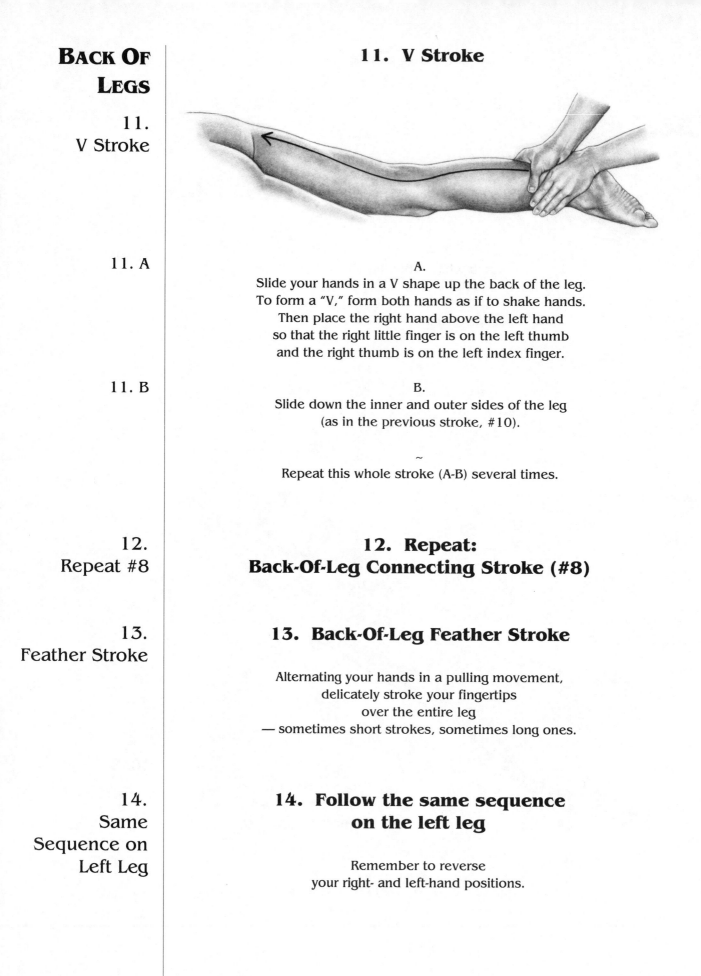

A.
Slide your hands in a V shape up the back of the leg.
To form a "V," form both hands as if to shake hands.
Then place the right hand above the left hand
so that the right little finger is on the left thumb
and the right thumb is on the left index finger.

B.
Slide down the inner and outer sides of the leg
(as in the previous stroke, #10).

~

Repeat this whole stroke (A-B) several times.

12. Repeat:
Back-Of-Leg Connecting Stroke (#8)

13. Back-Of-Leg Feather Stroke

Alternating your hands in a pulling movement,
delicately stroke your fingertips
over the entire leg
— sometimes short strokes, sometimes long ones.

14. Follow the same sequence
on the left leg

Remember to reverse
your right- and left-hand positions.

BACK SIDE CONCLUSION

15. Back Hug

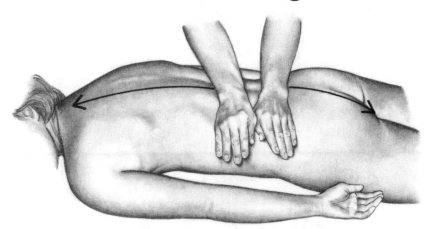

A.
(This may be a difficult stroke
unless you are using a massage table.)

Using the soft, inner side of your forearms,
begin at your lover's lower back
and slide them to below the buttocks
and to the upper back.

Then slide your forearms back together.
~
Repeat this whole movement several times.

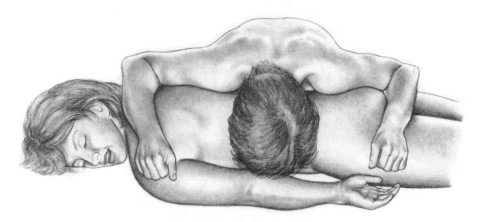

B.
After a few repetitions of Part A,
rest your chest on the back.

Be very careful
not to put pressure on the neck and throat area.

16. Concluding Stroke

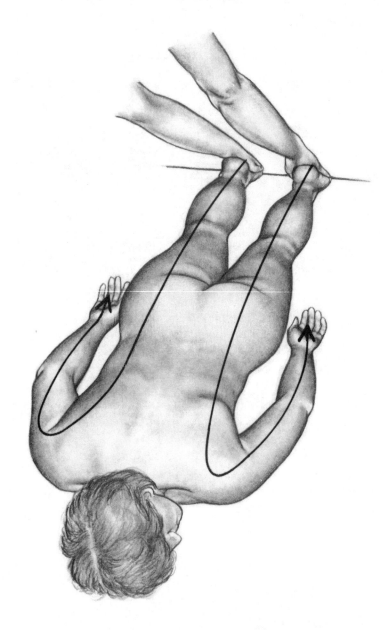

In one long movement, slowly slide your hands up
from the feet
to the shoulder
and off the fingertips.

If you wish, then gently feather stroke
with your fingertips
the entire back side.

~

After a while, with a gentle voice,
invite your lover to turn over when ready.

Instructions: Written as applied to the right arm.
Lover's Position: Lying on back with arms by side.
Your Position: Initially at the right waist, facing the head.

17. Connecting Stroke

17.
Connecting
Stroke

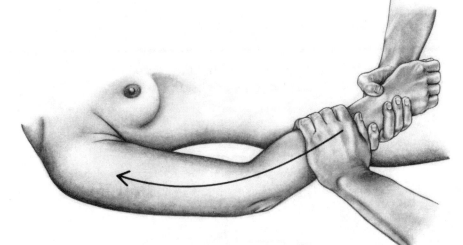

A.
First, gently hold the right wrist in your right hand.
Then with the little-finger side leading,
slide your left hand up
the outside of the right arm.

17. A

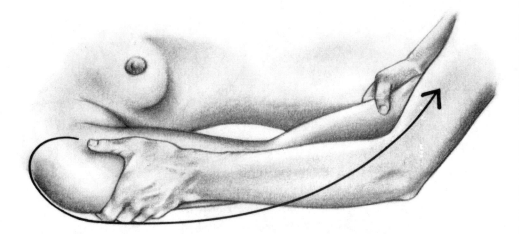

B.
Pivot on the shoulder tip
and slide down
on the back side of the arm.

17. B

Connecting
Stroke

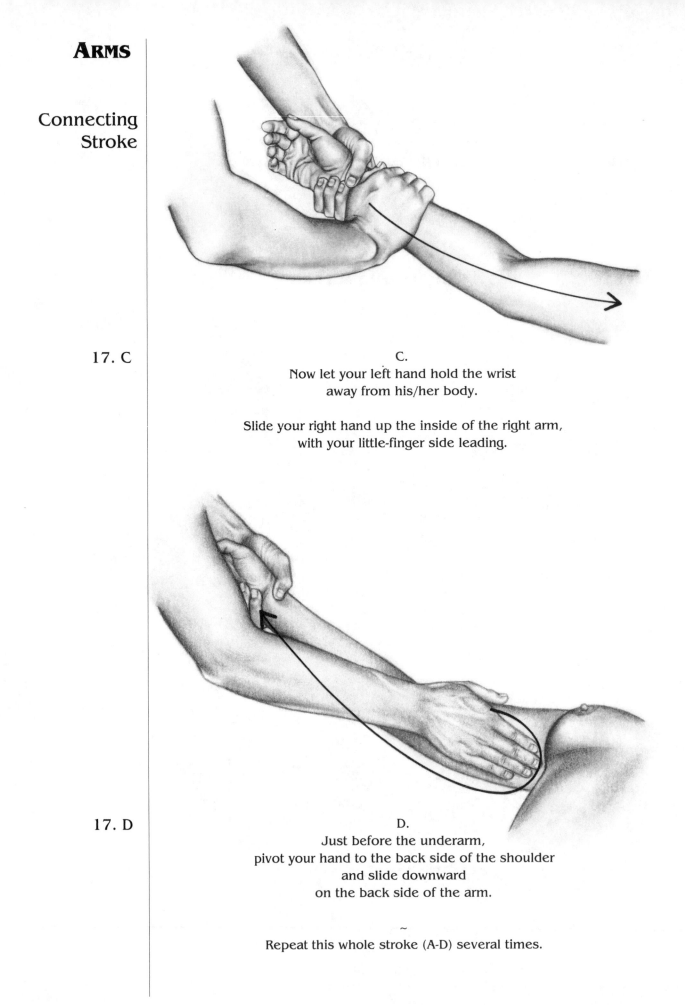

17. C

C.
Now let your left hand hold the wrist
away from his/her body.

Slide your right hand up the inside of the right arm,
with your little-finger side leading.

17. D

D.
Just before the underarm,
pivot your hand to the back side of the shoulder
and slide downward
on the back side of the arm.

~

Repeat this whole stroke (A-D) several times.

18. Upper Arm Stroke

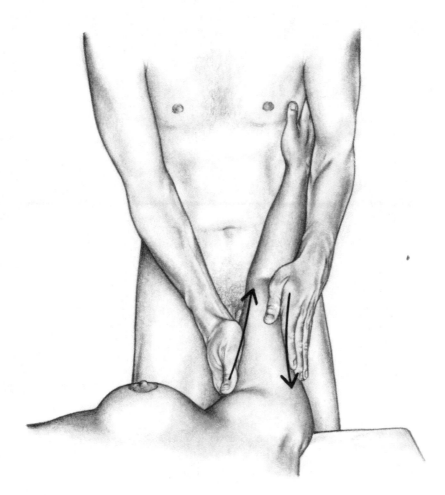

A.
Hold the right hand on your left rib cage.

Slide your left hand upward
on the outside of his/her upper arm

while your right hand slides downward
on the back side.

ARMS

Upper Arm
Stroke

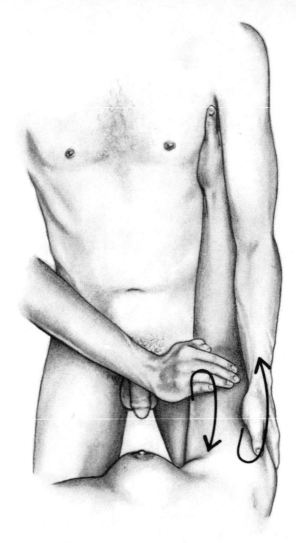

18. B

B.
Your left hand rotates on the shoulder
and slides downward
on the back side of the upper arm

while your right hand rotates at the elbow
and slides upward
on the upper side of the upper arm.

18. C

C.
Your left hand rotates at the elbow
and slides upward
on the outside of the upper arm
(which is Part A again)

while your right hand rotates at the underarm
and slides downward
on the back side
(which is Part A again).

~

Repeat this whole stroke (A-C) several times.

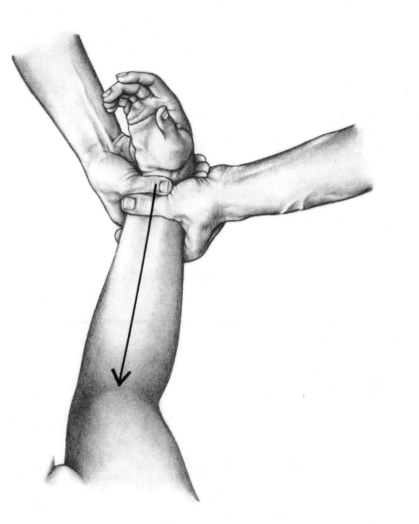

19. Forearm Stroke

A.
Holding the forearm upright,
slide the flat sides of your thumbs
down the inside of the forearm.
Let your thumbs be parallel with each other.

B.
When your thumbs reach the inner side of the elbow,
lighten your touch
and slide your hands back up to the wrist.

~

Continue with the right hand
before massaging the left arm.

20.
Hand Curl

HANDS

Instructions: Written as applied to the right hand.

20. Hand Curl

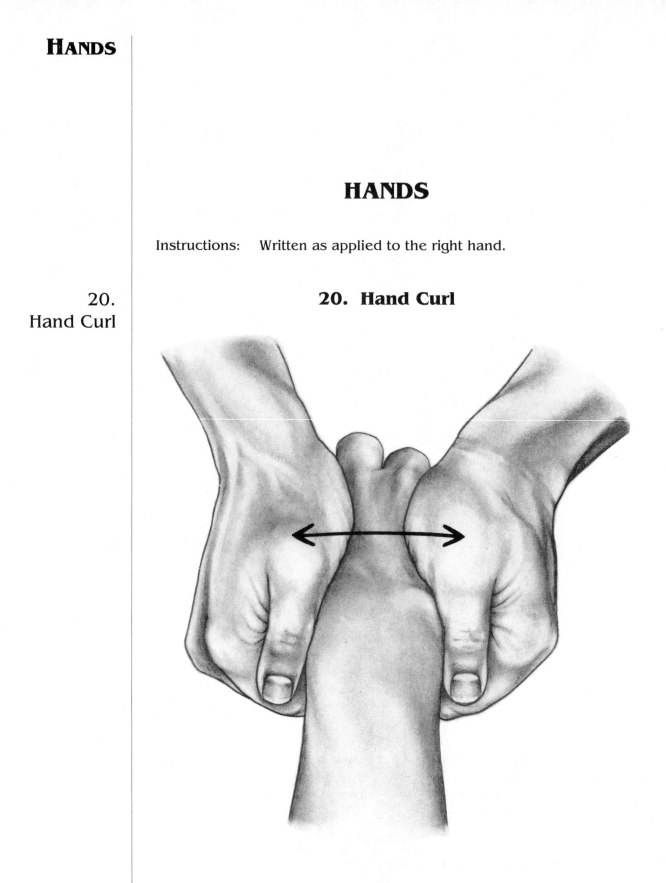

On the back side of the hand,
firmly slide the heels of your thumbs outward
to the sides of the hand
while curling the hand inward.
~
Repeat this stroke several times.

21. Palm Massage

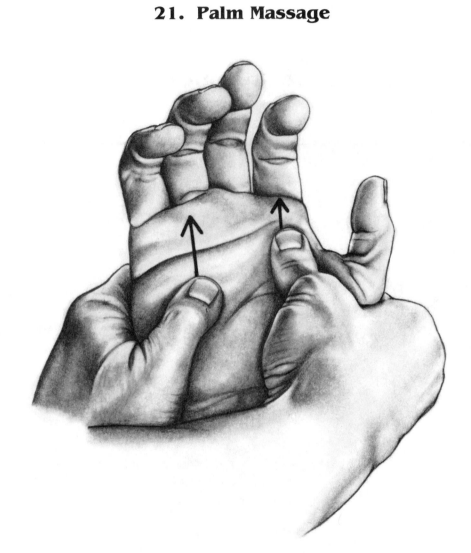

Alternating your thumbs,
firmly push your thumb pads upward on the palm.
Repeat the movements many times,
covering the palm entirely.

22.
Web Stroke

22. Web Stroke

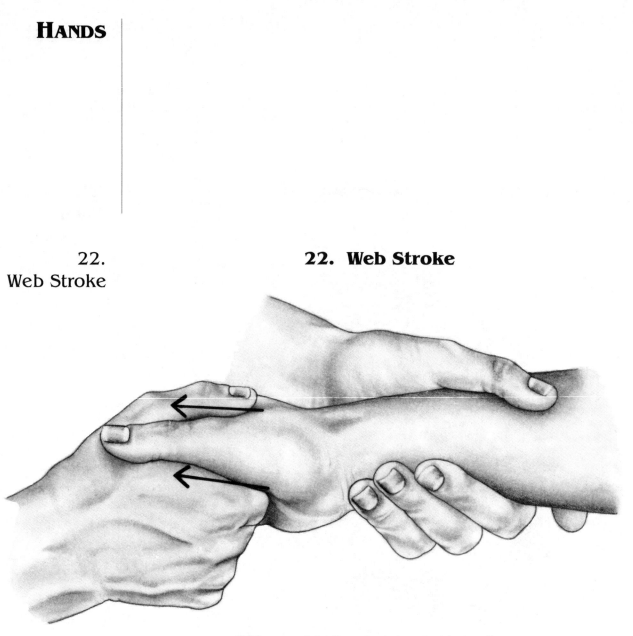

With your right thumb and curled index finger
between the right thumb and first finger,
slide outward firmly.

~

Repeat this stroke several times.

23. Finger Stroke

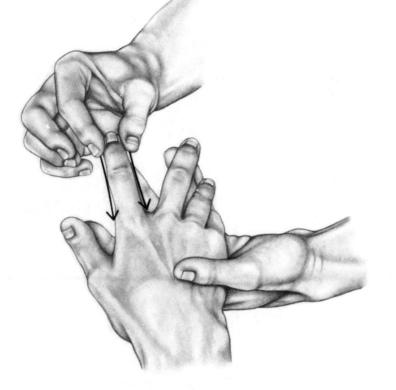

A.
Starting at the tip of the finger,
slide very lightly down the sides of the finger
with your thumb and finger
— very, very lightly.

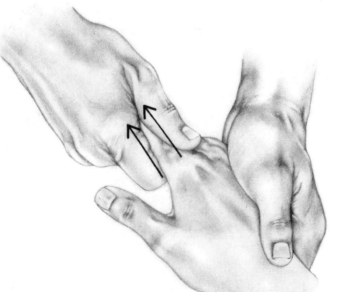

B.
Grasping the finger firmly at its base,
slide up and off the finger.

~

Repeat Part A and Part B once on the thumb
and once on each finger.

24. Palm Reading

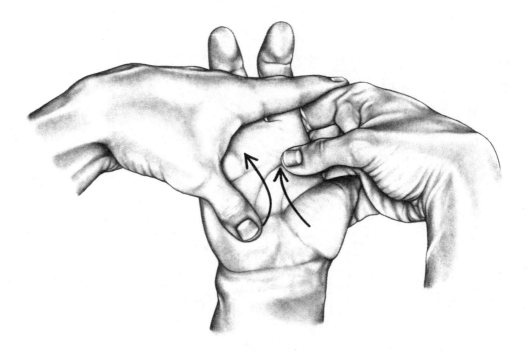

Interlacing your fingers with your lover's,
stretch the palm open
and lightly feather stroke the palm
with your thumb tips
— very, very, very lightly.

25. Repeat: Arm Connecting Stroke (#17)

26. Arm and Hand Feather Stroke

Alternating your hands in a pulling movement,
delicately stroke your fingertips
over the entire arm and hand
— sometimes short strokes, sometimes long ones.

27. Follow the same Arm and Hand sequence on the left arm

Remember to reverse
your right- and left-hand positions.

FRONT OF LEGS

Instructions: Written as applied to the right leg.

28. Connecting Stroke

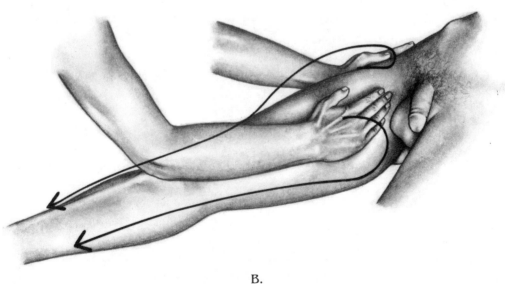

A.
With your left hand in front,
slide your hands up the front of the leg.

(For both hands, the little-finger-side leads;
the thumbs are beside their index fingers.)

B.
Near the pelvis, rotate your hands outward
and slide down the inner and outer sides of the leg.

~

Repeat this whole stroke (A-B) several times.

29.
Mini-
Connecting
Stroke

29. Mini-Connecting Stroke

On the thigh,
make a series of connecting strokes
similar to the previous stroke (#28)
but shorter and only on the thigh.

Each succeeding stroke starts
a little farther up the thigh
and ends a little farther up.

~

Repeat this whole series several times.

30. Thigh Kneading

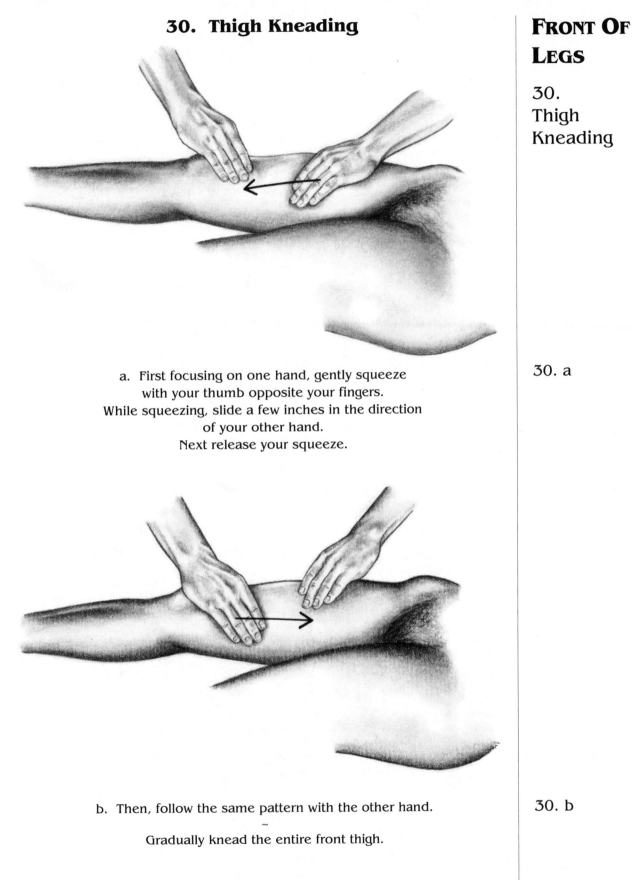

a. First focusing on one hand, gently squeeze
with your thumb opposite your fingers.
While squeezing, slide a few inches in the direction
of your other hand.
Next release your squeeze.

b. Then, follow the same pattern with the other hand.

~

Gradually knead the entire front thigh.

31. Repeat:
Front-Of-Leg Connecting Stroke (#28)

~

Continue with the right foot
before massaging the left leg.

32.
Ankle Circling

FEET

Instructions: Written as applied to the right foot.

32. Ankle Circling

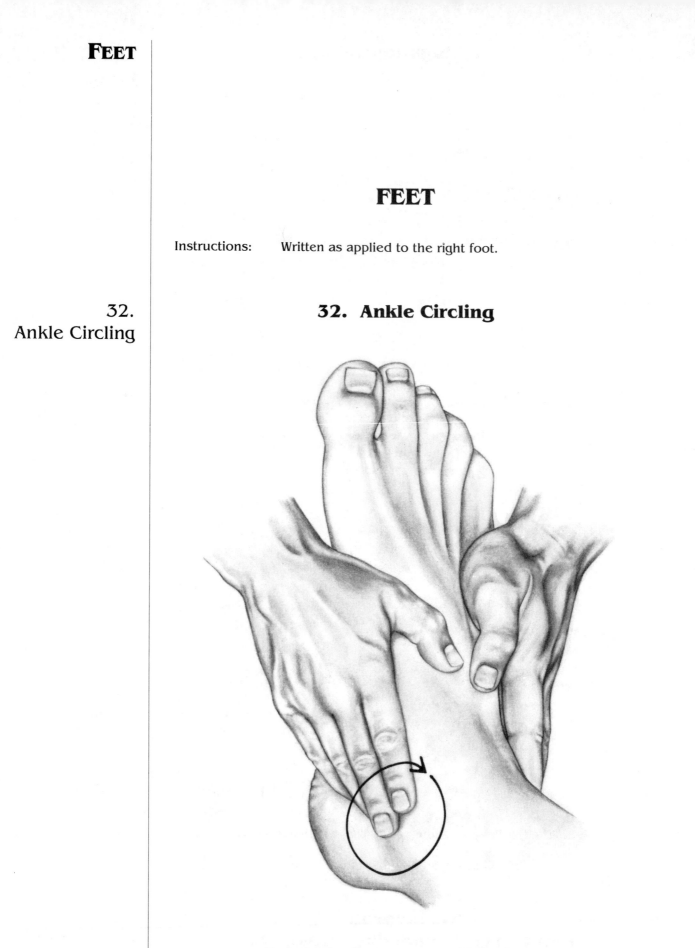

Stroke in circular movements with flat fingers
around the ankle.

33. Connecting Stroke

Alternating your hands,
squeeze the foot
and slide off the end.

~

Repeat this stroke several times.

34. Arc de Triomphe

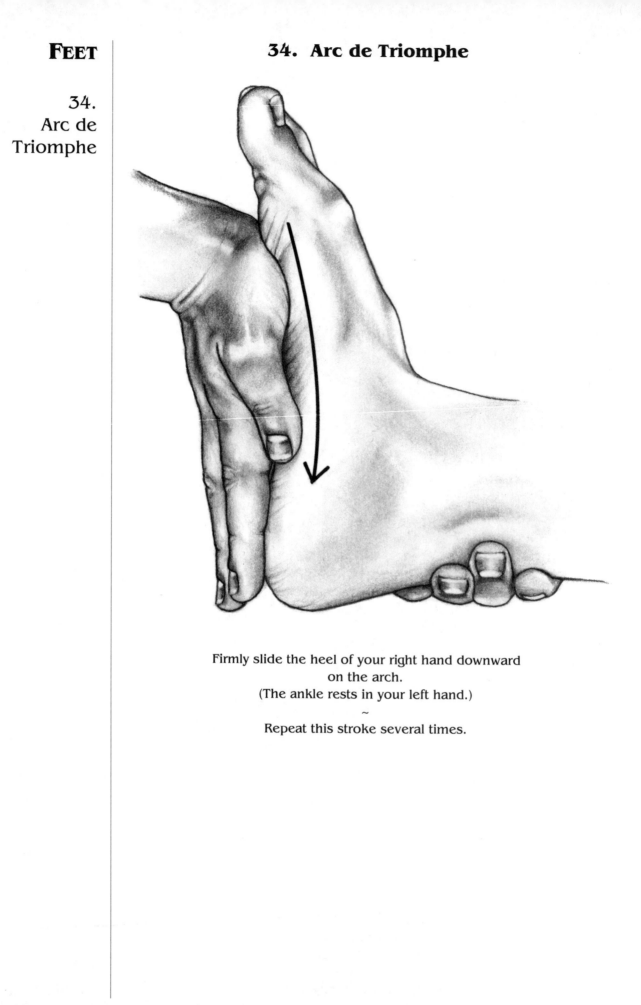

Firmly slide the heel of your right hand downward
on the arch.
(The ankle rests in your left hand.)

~

Repeat this stroke several times.

35. Finger Circles

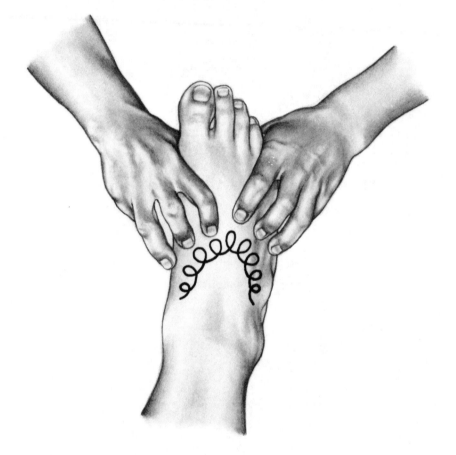

On the top of the foot,
make small circles with your finger pads.

(Slide your fingers over the skin
and/or, with a little more pressure,
slide your lover's skin over the muscles,
tendons, and bones beneath.)

~

Repeat these circles over the entire top of the foot.

36. Between-The-Toes Stroke

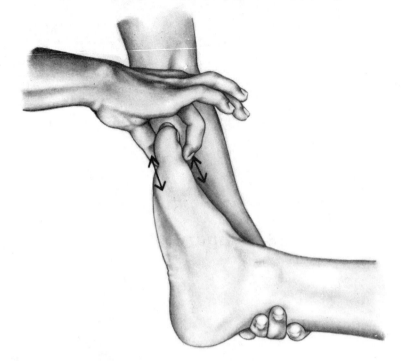

With your right-hand index finger
on top on the right foot
and your right-hand thumb on the bottom,
squeeze and slide up and down several times
between each of the toes.

37. Slithering

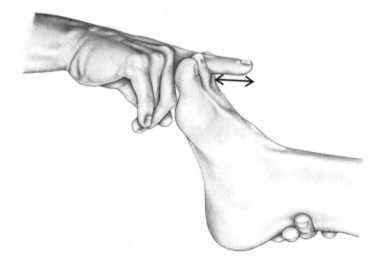

Very slowly and gently "screw" any right finger in and out
between each set of toes.

38. Repeat:
Front-Of-Leg Connecting Stroke (#28)

38.
Repeat #28

39. Leg and Foot Feather Stroke

Alternating your hands in a pulling movement,
delicately stroke your fingertips
over the entire leg and foot
— sometimes short strokes, sometimes long ones.

39.
Feather Stroke

40. Follow the same Front-Of-Legs and Feet sequence on the left side

~

Remember to reverse
your right- and left-hand positions.

40.
Same Front-Of-Legs and Feet Sequence on Left Side

FRONT TORSO

Your Position: Initially at your lover's right side.

41. Moon Stroke

First, practice your right- and left-hand movements separately:

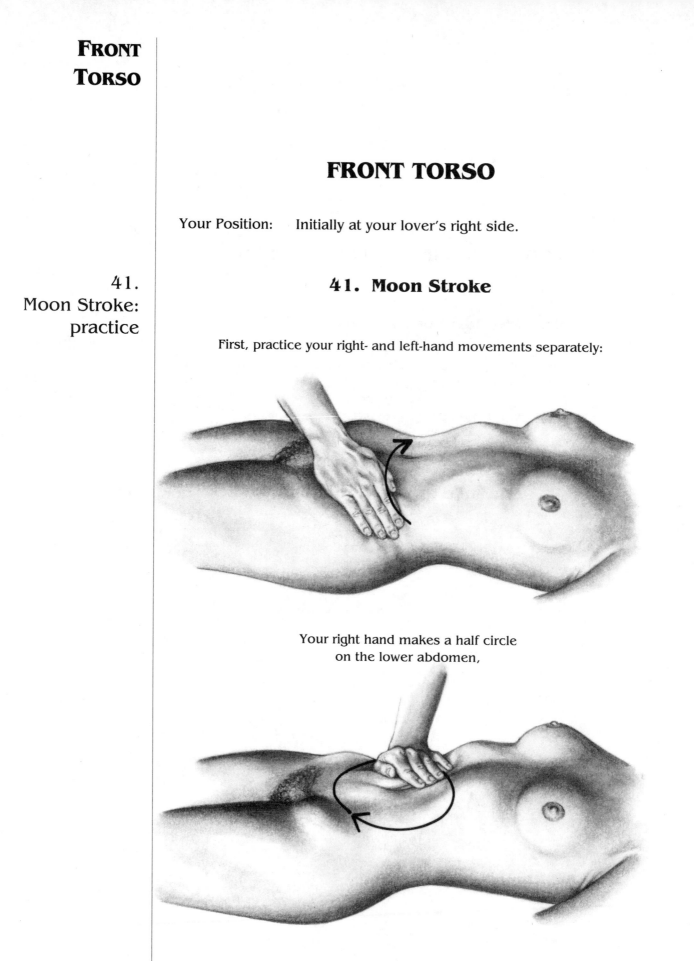

Your right hand makes a half circle
on the lower abdomen,

while your left hand makes a full circle
around the whole abdomen.

This is the complete version:

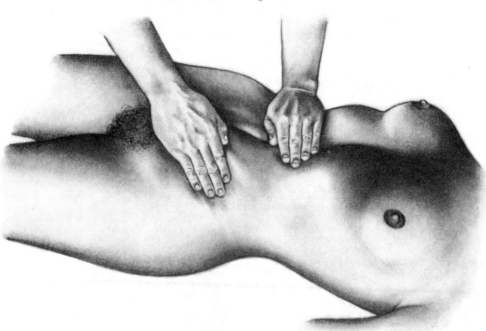

Coordinate your hand movements:
when your right hand is stroking in a half circle,
your left hand is directly opposite on the circle.

When not using your right hand,
simply lift it out of the way
of your left hand's full-circle pattern.
~
Repeat this whole stroke several times.

42. Center Slide

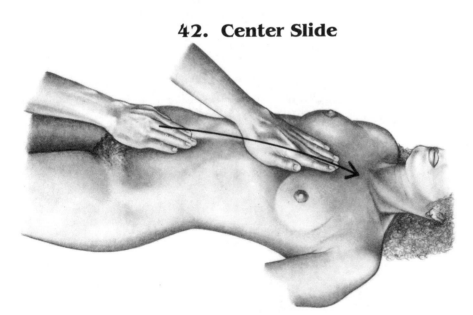

Alternating your hands,
firmly and slowly slide them up the midline
from the lower abdomen to the upper chest.

43. Breast Kneading

Instructions: Written as applied to the right breast.

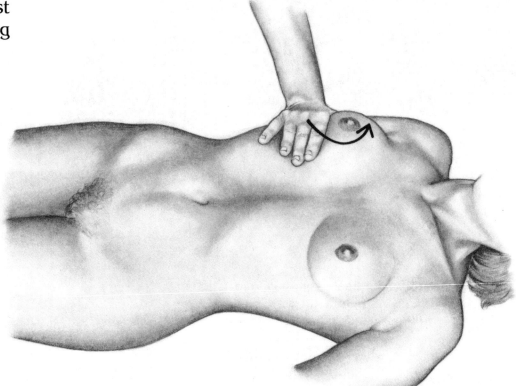

43. A

A.
Starting at the lower, outer side of the breast area,
slide your right hand up over the breast
so that your thumb and index finger
encircle the nipple.

Using the nipple as the axis,
continue the stroke
by rotating your hand counterclockwise
around the nipple
as you slide up and off the breast.

Breast
Kneading

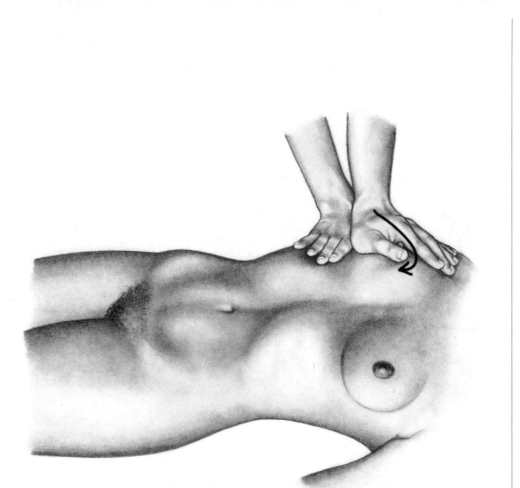

43. B

B.
Slide your left hand
from the same lower, outer side of the breast area
up over the breast
so that your thumb and index finger
encircle the nipple.

Using the nipple as the axis,
continue the stroke
by rotating your left hand clockwise
around the nipple
as you slide up and off the breast.

~
Repeat this series (A-B) several times
with one hand following the other.

~
Continue with the following stroke (#44)
on the right breast
before massaging the left breast.

Note:
On a woman's breast, apply a lighter pressure.

44. Spokes Stroke

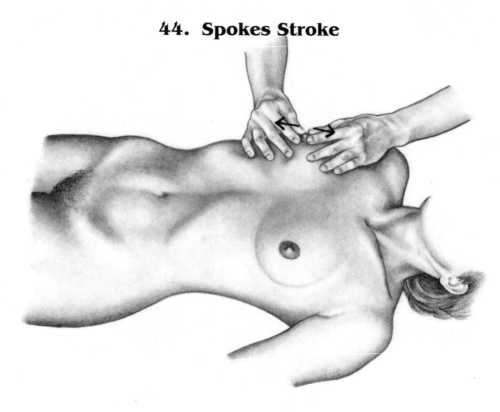

44. A

A.
Imagine the nipple as the axis in a wheel
with spokes radiating out from the axis.
Using the pads of the fingers and thumbs
of both hands,
gently squeeze at the axis
and slide out along a spoke,
moving your hands in opposite directions.

~

Repeat this pattern several times
along the different spokes.

44. B

B.
Gently squeeze the base of the nipple
between the pads
of your index finger and thumb
of one hand
and slide UP and off the nipple.
Follow this pattern,
alternating your hands
one immediately after the other.

~

Now move to the other side
and repeat this and the previous stroke
(#43 and #44)
on the other breast area.

45. Side Pulling

A.
Alternating your hands,
slide them in a pulling manner
across the side of the torso
toward the front midline.

~

(This series includes the area
from the hips to near the underarms.
Be gentle on the mammary area.)

B.
Move to the other side,
and apply the pulling movements
to the opposite side.

46. Torso Feather Stroke

Alternating your hands in a pulling movement,
delicately stroke your fingertips
over the entire torso.
Include the genital and thigh areas as well.

GENITALS: MALE

Lover's Position: Lying on back.
Your Position: To your lover's right side.
Note: If you wish to follow safer-sex practices, please consult the appendix.

47.
Anointing With
Oil

47. Anointing With Oil

47. A

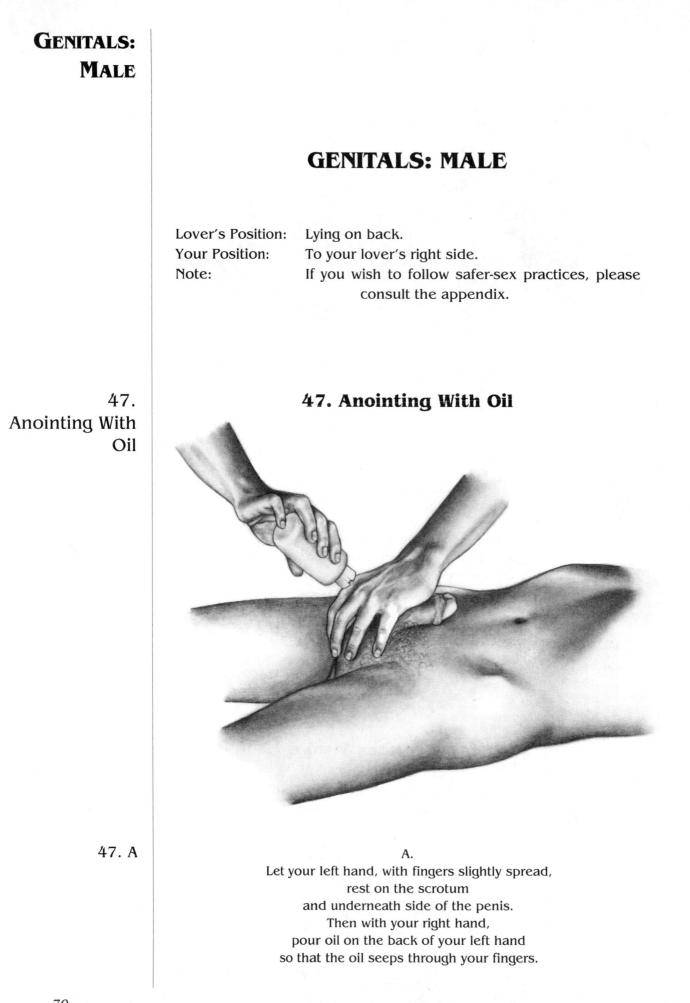

A.
Let your left hand, with fingers slightly spread,
rest on the scrotum
and underneath side of the penis.
Then with your right hand,
pour oil on the back of your left hand
so that the oil seeps through your fingers.

Anointing With
Oil

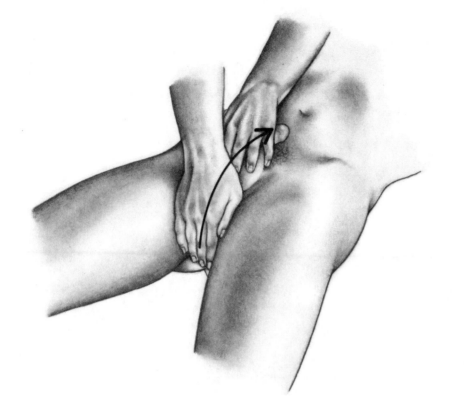

B.
Alternating your hands,
spread the oil with a pulling up motion,
sliding from the pelvic floor up
over the scrotum and penis.

Perhaps give a little firmer pressure
on the pelvic floor.

Be sure there is plenty of oil
since the following strokes
assume well-lubricated motions.

~

Note: Should your lover ejaculate during this or any other stroke
perhaps go to "Being," #58.

47. B

48.
The Coronal
Stroke

48. The Coronal Stroke

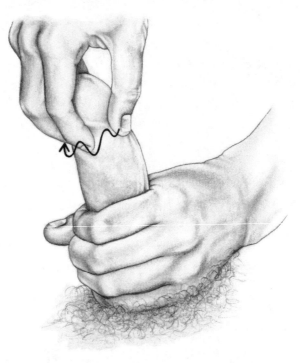

Your left hand gently stretches the foreskin down
along the shaft of the flaccid or erect penis.

Your right hand points
as if to twist a halved orange on a juicer.
Concentrating on the head of the penis,
rotate your right-hand fingers back and forth
in coordination with an up-and-down sliding motion.

Vary the amount of pressure from your right hand.

49. The Serpent

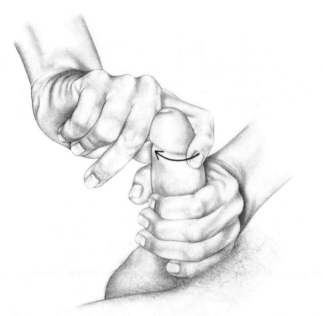

a: Your left hand gently stretches the foreskin down
along the shaft of the flaccid or erect penis.

Your right thumb and index finger form a snug circle
just below the head of the penis
and rotate in a clockwise direction
as far as your wrist permits.

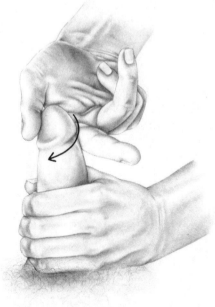

b: Continuing the movement, lift your right thumb
so that your index finger can maintain
contact in the rotation
until the thumb can form a circle
with the index finger again.

~

Repeat this circling several times.

50. The Ten Stroke

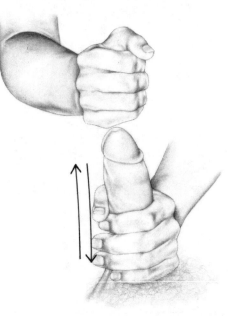

Using plenty of oil and alternating your hands,
make ten downward strokes
on the flaccid or erect penis,
then ten upward strokes.
Follow with nine downward, nine upward,
eight downward, eight upward
—all the way to one down and one up.

~

Suggestion:
syncopate the rhythm of your stroking.
Rather than using an even beat (1-2-3-4-5-6),
wait a moment after each set of two strokes
(1-2—3-4—5-6).

51. The Scrotum Ring

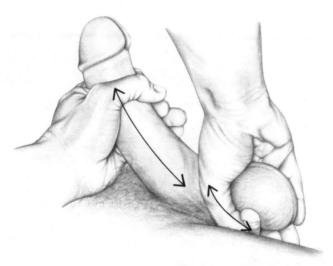

Your right thumb along with your index
and perhaps middle fingers
encircle the scrotum
between the base of the penis and the testicles.
(Be careful not to squeeze the testicles.)

Now move the scrotum up and down
as your left hand strokes up and down
on the flaccid or erect penile shaft.

Vary the amount of pressure of your right hand
against the base of the penis.
~
To continue the Male Genital strokes,
go to "Inner Connections," #57,
which is for both men and women.

GENITALS: FEMALE

Lover's Position: Lying on back.
Your Position: To your lover's right side.
Note: Be certain your fingernails are smooth and short
        and your hands are clean
        when massaging membranous tissues areas.
Note: If you wish to follow safer-sex practices,
        please consult the appendix.

52.
Anointing With
Oil

52. Anointing With Oil

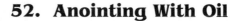

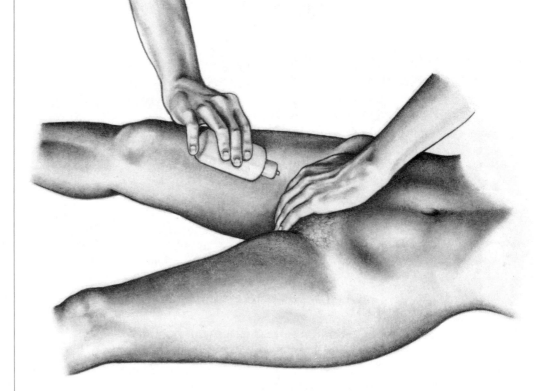

52. A

A.
Let your left hand, with fingers slightly spread,
rest on the vulva.
Then with your right hand,
pour the lubricant or oil
on the back of your left hand
so that the lubricant or oil
seeps through your fingers.

Anointing With
Oil

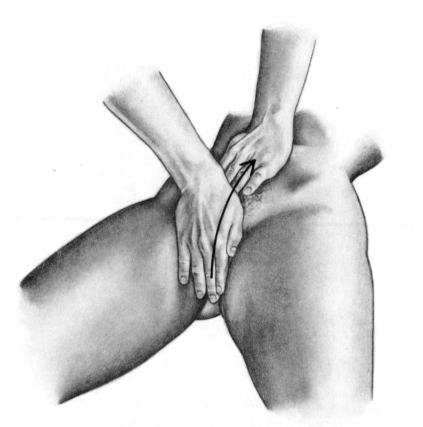

B.
Alternating your hands,
spread the lubricant or oil with a pulling up motion
by sliding from the lower part of the vulva
up over the clitoris and pubic area.

~

Note:
Be very careful not to stroke
from the anal to the vaginal areas.

52. B

53. The Vulva Stroke

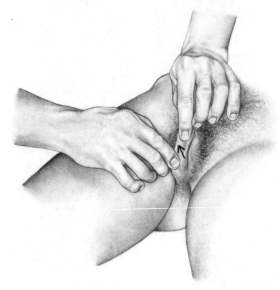

This is a series of strokes on each outer and inner lip.
With a thumb on one side of a lip
and the index finger on the other side,
very gently squeeze and slide off the edge of the lip.

Alternating your hands, continue this pattern
along the entire length of each lip.

54. The Clitoris Stroke

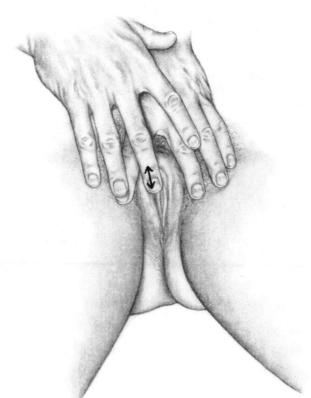

A.
Now you center your stroking
around the head of the clitoris,
which is just beneath where the inner lips
merge together at the upper part of the vulva.

To begin,
slide the middle finger pad of your right hand
up and down several times
between the inner and outer lips
on one side of the vulva
and then on the other side.

54. A

B.
With one or two fingers, slowly massage circles
around the clitoral head,
several times in one directions,
then several times in the other direction.

54. B

C.
With a single finger pad,
begin a very slow, upward stroke
at the vaginal entrance,
up through the inner lips, up past the clitoral head.
Repeat several times.

54. C

55. The Clock

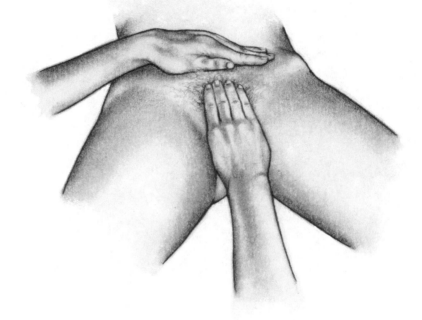

55. A

A.
For this intravaginal massage,
imagine a clock at the vaginal entrance,
with twelve o'clock near the clitoris
and six o'clock near the anus.

Your left palm rests on the abdomen.

At the twelve-o'clock position
slowly introduce your right thumb
into the vagina
until its pad is pressing upward
on the underneath side
of the pubic bone.

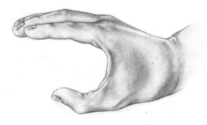

Now gently rock your right arm and hand
back and forth about an inch.

After about fifteen seconds or longer,
lighten your pressure,
slide your thumb to the one-o'clock position,
and begin to rock again.
Continue in this fashion
until about the seven-o'clock position.

The Clock

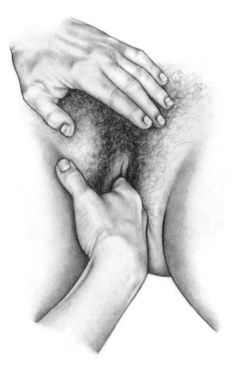

B.
At about seven o'clock,
shift to using your index finger
and continue with the rocking pattern
up through twelve o'clock.

55. B

56. The G-Spot Stroke

A.
This stroke may be easier
if you bring your lover's knees up
with both feet resting on the table.

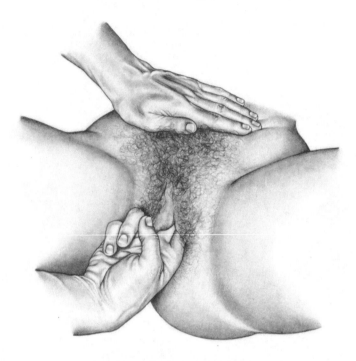

Your left palm rests on the abdomen.

At the twelve-o'clock position
slowly introduce
your right index and middle fingers
into the vagina
until the finger pads are pressing
upward
above (beyond) the pubic bone.
(This is approximately
the G-Spot area
inside the vagina.)

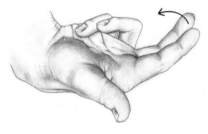

Here make a "come here" finger movement
to stroke your finger pads
across the membranous tissue.
Vary the pressure to find what feels best
— if there is pain,
lighten the pressure or discontinue the stroking.

The G-Spot
Stroke

B.
With your right hand continuing Part A,
rest the heel of your left hand on the lower abdomen.
Now allow your left-hand fingers to delicately stroke the clitoral head
at the same time.

(Perhaps apply a little pressure
on the lower abdomen
with the heel of your left hand.)

When you complete the stroke,
slide your lover's legs back to the flat position.

56. B

Note: Starting with this stroke, the male and female genital massage description is the same.

57. Inner Connections

In this series of strokes
you connect the enjoyable sensations of the genitals
with the enjoyable sensations
of other parts of the body.

57.
Inner
Connections

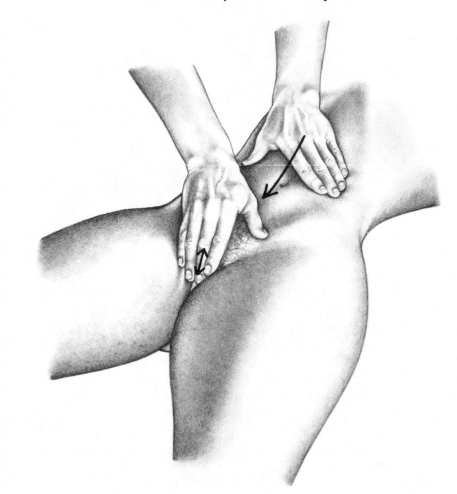

57. A

A. Abdomen and Genitals

While your right hand massages the genitals
(in any fashion)
let your left hand knead
or make circular strokes on the abdomen
(For a description of kneading, see stroke #9.)

Inner
Connections

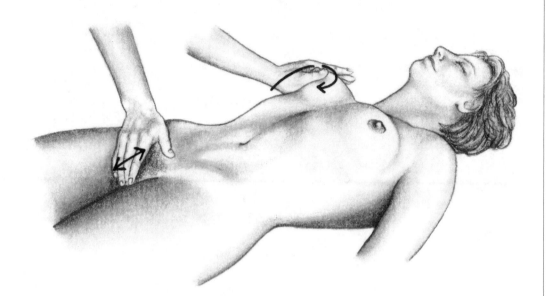

B. Breast Area and Genitals

57. B

As your right hand continues as in Part A,
slide your left hand from the same lower, outer side of the breast area
up over the breast
so that your thumb and index finger
encircle the nipple.
Using the nipple as the axis,
continue the stroke
by rotating your left hand clockwise
around the nipple
as you slide up and off the breast.
~
Repeat several times on the right breast area
and continue Part C on the right side of the neck
before going to the left side.

Inner
Connections

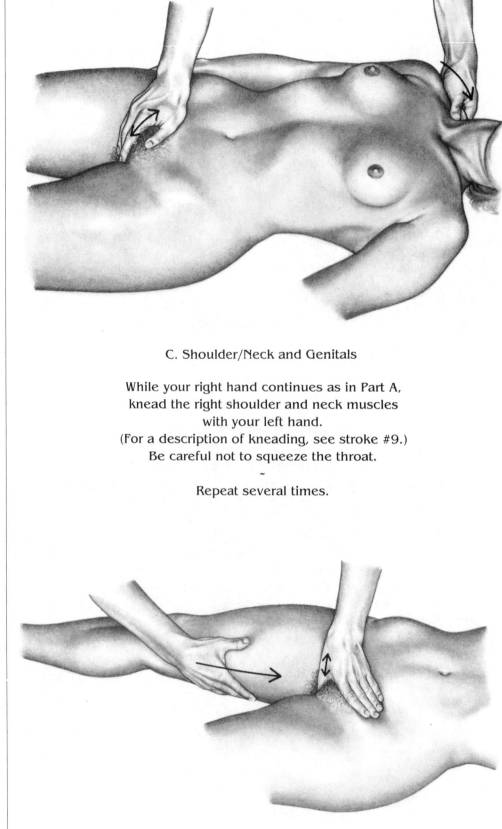

57. C

C. Shoulder/Neck and Genitals

While your right hand continues as in Part A,
knead the right shoulder and neck muscles
with your left hand.
(For a description of kneading, see stroke #9.)
Be careful not to squeeze the throat.

~

Repeat several times.

57. D

D. Inner Thigh and Genitals

Now your hands change positions:
your left sliding down to massage the genitals
while your right kneads the right inner thigh.

Inner
Connections

57. E

E. Change Sides

If it is possible, move to the other side
and follow the same sequence
while simply reversing
the left-hand and right-hand instructions.
(If you cannot easily move to the over side,
modify your stroking so that the left breast,
neck/shoulder, and thigh areas are massaged also.)

Once you complete this series,
move back to your lover's right side
for the following instructions.
(Remember to keep hand contact if possible.)

58.
Being

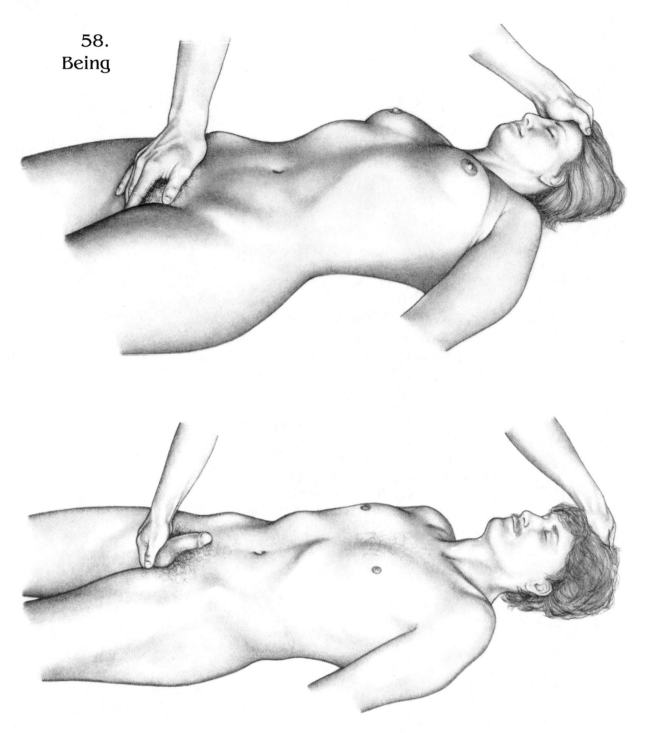

58. A

A.
Rest your left hand on the head
so that your palm is on the forehead
and your fingers are on the center top of the head.

At the other end of an imaginary axis
through the core of the body,
rest your right hand on the pelvic area
so that your palm is on the vulva,
or the scrotum if you are massaging a man.

(58. A continued)

Now give a soft verbal invitation to your beloved
to take a slightly fuller inhalation
and to imagine the breath
beginning at the floor of his/her pelvis
and coming up the core of the body
to the top of his/her head.

Then for the exhalation,
invite your beloved to simply let go of the breath
and to imagine the breath reversing
and flowing from the top of the head
down through the core of the body
and out the floor of the pelvis.

~

Continue this breathing and imaging guidance
for perhaps two to five minutes.

~

Here we are focusing directly
on the subtle energy bodies.
In the pelvic floor area is
the first, or Muladhara, chakra.
At the top of the head is
the crown, or Sahasrara, chakra.

Often the genital massage
stimulates sexual feelings,
turns on the generator in the pelvic area.
This laying on of hands, Being,
encourages the expansion of energy
throughout the body.

This is the shift
from friction sex
to tantric sex.

Being

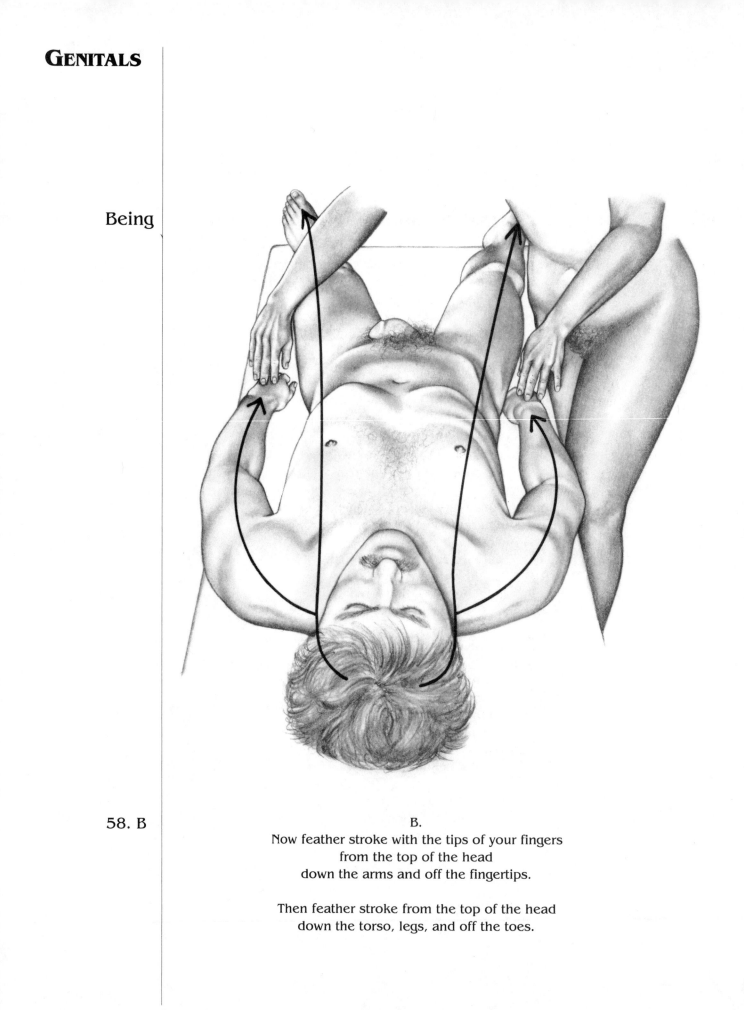

58. B

B.
Now feather stroke with the tips of your fingers
from the top of the head
down the arms and off the fingertips.

Then feather stroke from the top of the head
down the torso, legs, and off the toes.

Being

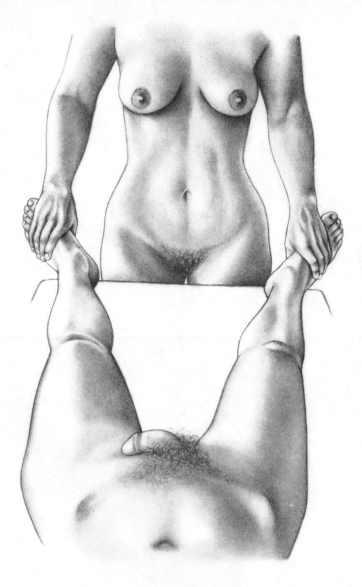

58. C

C.
Now rest your hands on the feet
with your thumbs on the arches
and your fingers on top of the feet.

Here again softly give breathing
and imaging instructions:
the inhalation comes from the bottom of the feet
up to the top of the head
The exhalation flows from the top of the head
down to the bottom of the feet.

After a couple of minutes
gradually allow your hands to ascend,
up off your beloved's feet.

NECK AND HEAD

Your Position: Behind the head.

59.
Connecting
Stroke

59. A

59. Connecting Stroke

A.
Place your left hand
on the left side of the head
so that your thumb is
in front of the ear
and the fingers
are behind the ear.

Then rotate the head
toward the left shoulder.

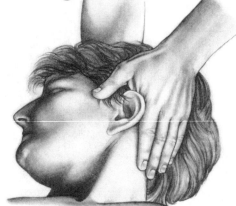

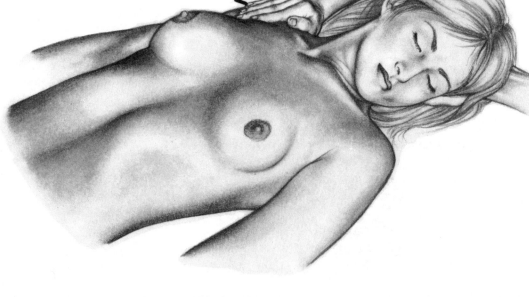

59. B

B.
Place your right palm on the right shoulder
and stretch downward.

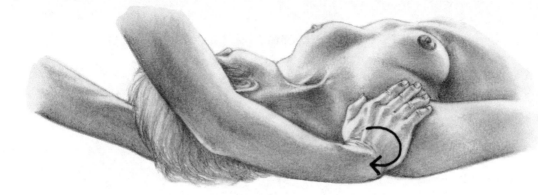

C.
Discontinue the stretching
and pivot your hand outward on the shoulder.

D.
Firmly slide the flat of your fingers upward
on the back of the neck
(not on the throat).

~

Repeat steps B, C, and D several times
and then follow the same sequence
on the other side of the neck,
reversing the instructions
for your right and left hands.

60. Let The Fingers Do The Walking

With the head resting on
the heels of your palms,
"walk" the finger pads
upward
on the back of the neck.

The "walking" is a sliding movement
of alternating fingers
from the base of the neck
toward the bottom of the skull.
(Use a firm pressure with your fingers,
but be careful not to pull the hair.)

61. Head Scratch

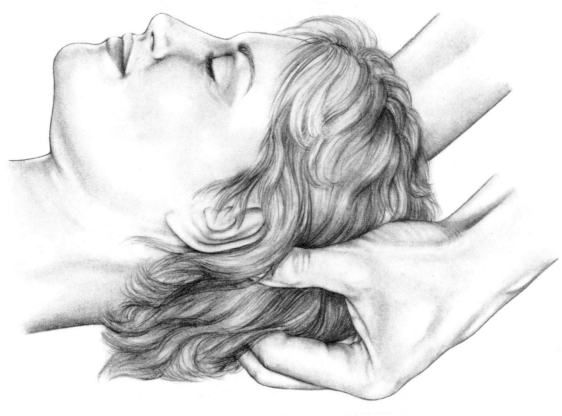

61. A

A.
Slide your finger pads back and forth
across the scalp on the underneath side of the head.

Head Scratch

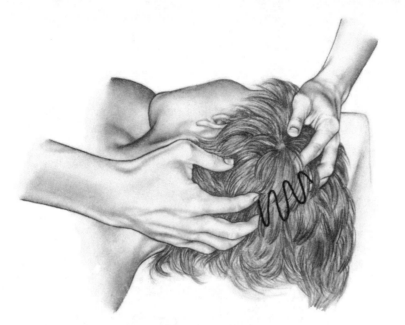

B.
Move to the right side
and turn your lover's face to the right.
Slide your finger pads back and forth across the scalp
on the left side of the head.

61. B

C.
Move to the left side and turn the face to the left.
Slide your finger pads back and forth across the scalp
on the right side of the head.

61. C

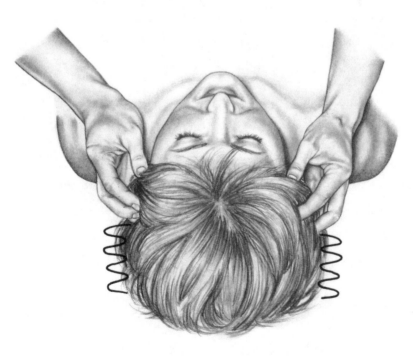

D.
Remain on the left side and turn the face upward.
Slide your finger pads back and forth
across the scalp on the sides and top of the head.

Gradually quicken the speed (but not the pressure).

61. D

E.
Without slowing down,
suddenly lift your fingers off the head.

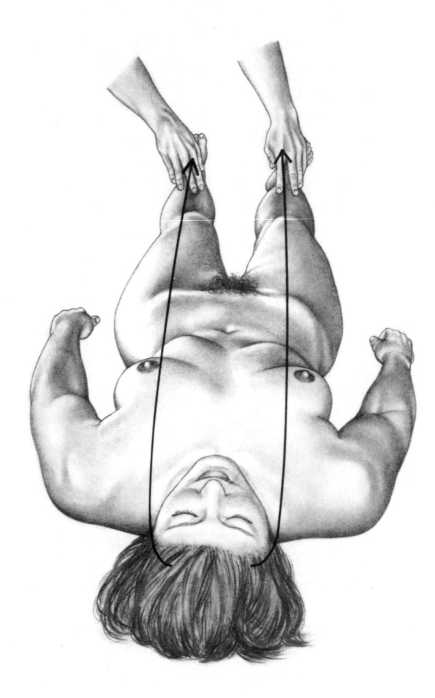

61. F

F.
Wait a few moments, and then if possible,
give a light feather stroke with your fingertips
from the head down and off the toes.

FACE

Your Position: Behind the head.

Note: It is best not to apply more oil for a facial massage. However, if you
         have been using an unscented oil, you might try a small
         drop of scented oil.

62. T Stroke

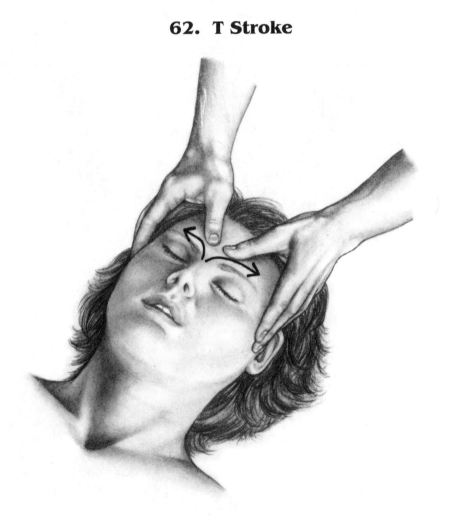

Slide your thumbs up and across the brow.
Three or four repetitions
will probably cover the whole brow.

63.
Eyebrow
Squeeze

63. Eyebrow Squeeze

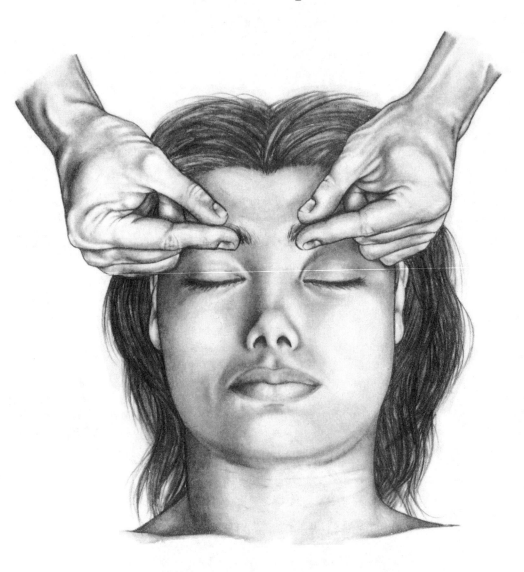

Make a series of squeezes of the eyebrows
from the midline outward.

64. Temple Circles

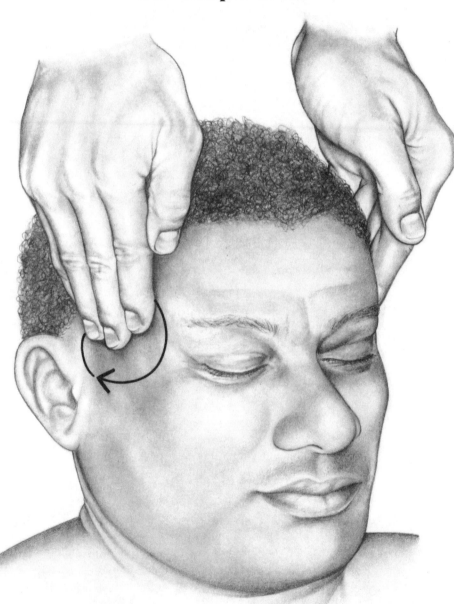

Make circle movements on the temples
with flat fingers.
Apply enough pressure
so his/her skin slides over the muscles beneath.

65.
Underneath-
The-Eyes
Stroke

65. Underneath-The-Eyes Stroke

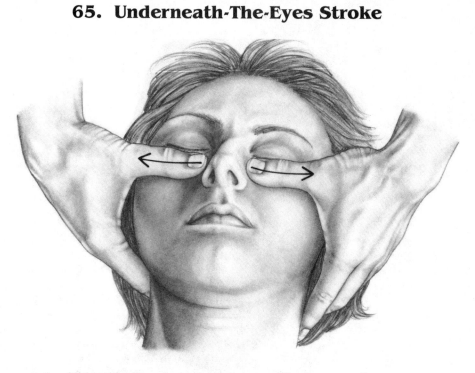

Slide your thumbs outward across the bony surface
underneath the eyes.

66.
Eye Stroke

66. Eye Stroke

Massage the eyes only if hard contact lens
have been removed;
light pressure on soft lens may be OK.

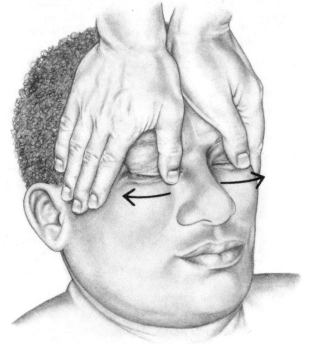

Bracing the heel of your thumbs on the forehead,
slowly slide your thumb pads
outward across the closed eyes.
Repeat two or three times.

67. Cheek Bone Stroke

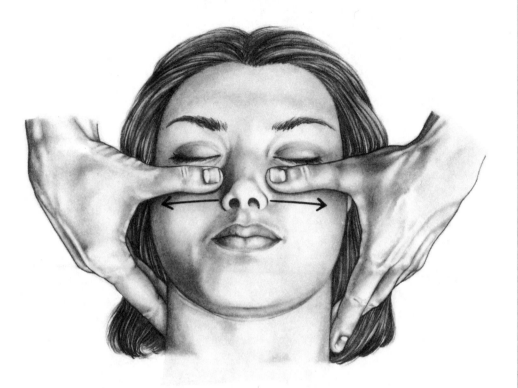

Slide your thumbs outward
across the top of the cheek bone.

68. Under-The-Cheek-Bone Stroke

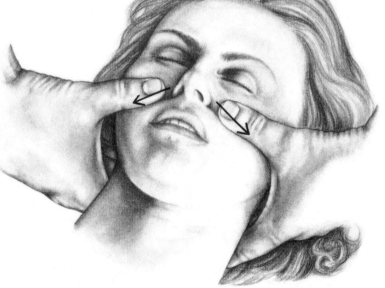

Slide your thumbs outward
underneath the cheek bone.

69.
Jaw Circles

69. Jaw Circles

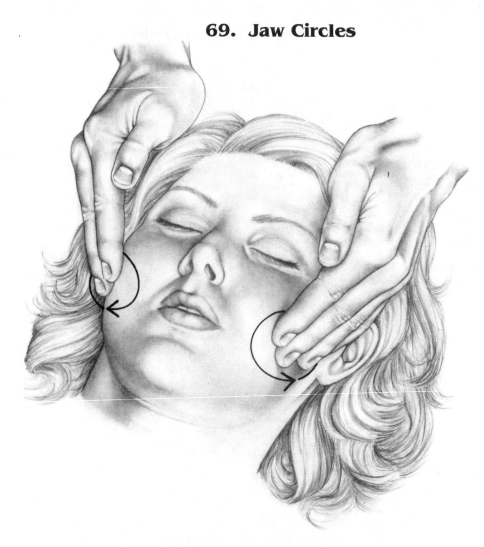

Make circle movements on the jaw area
with flat fingers.
Apply enough pressure
so his/her skin slides over the muscles beneath.

70.
Upper Lip
Stroke

70. Upper Lip Stroke

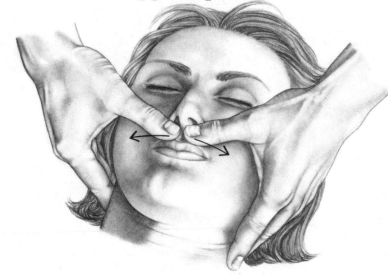

Slide your thumbs outward across the upper lip.

71. Lower Lip Stroke

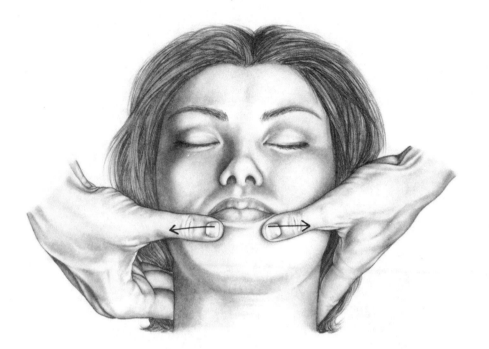

Slide your thumbs outward across the lower lip.

72. Throat Stroke

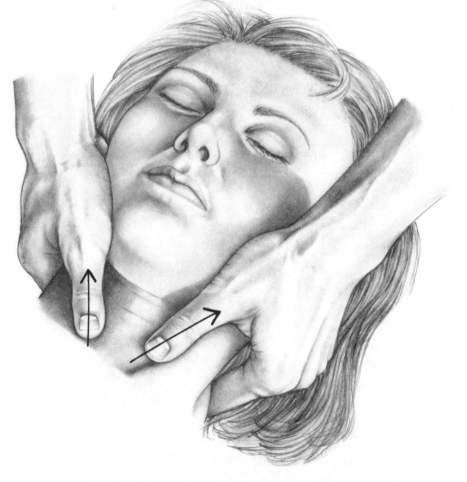

Slide your thumbs upward along the groove
between the larynx and the sides of the throat.

73. Behind-The-Ear Stroke

73.
Behind-The-Ear
Stroke

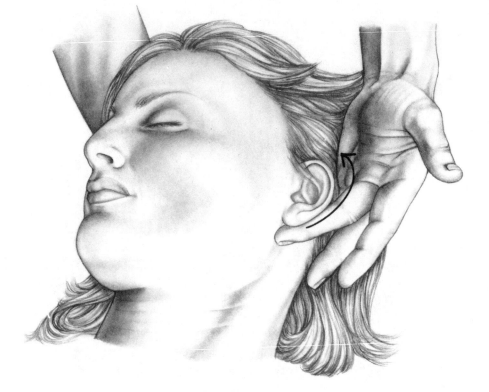

Slide your middle fingers
up and down along the grooves
behind the ears.

74.
Outer Ear
Stroke

74. Outer Ear Stroke

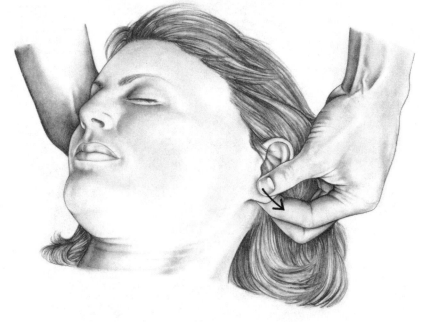

Gently squeeze the ear lobes
and slide outward to the edges.

~

Repeat this along the entire outer ear surface.

75. Inner Peace

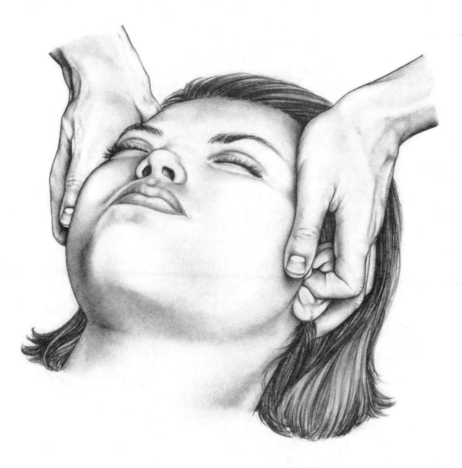

A.
Slowly slide your fingers into the ear canals
and relax in this position for about a minute,
blocking out the external sounds.

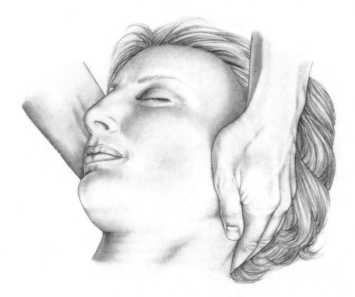

B.
If Part A is difficult for you
or uncomfortable for your lover,
cover the ears with your cupped palms.

CONCLUSION

76. Concluding Stroke

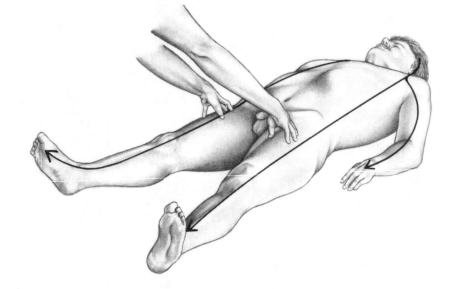

With your fingertips,
lightly feather stroke from the top of the head
down off the fingertips.
Then lightly feather stroke from the top of the head
down off the toes.

77. Covering

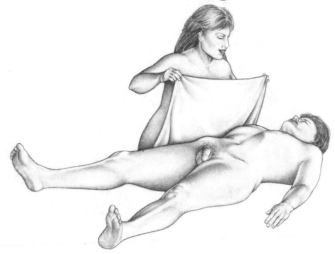

Unless it is very warm,
cover your beloved with a towel or sheet.

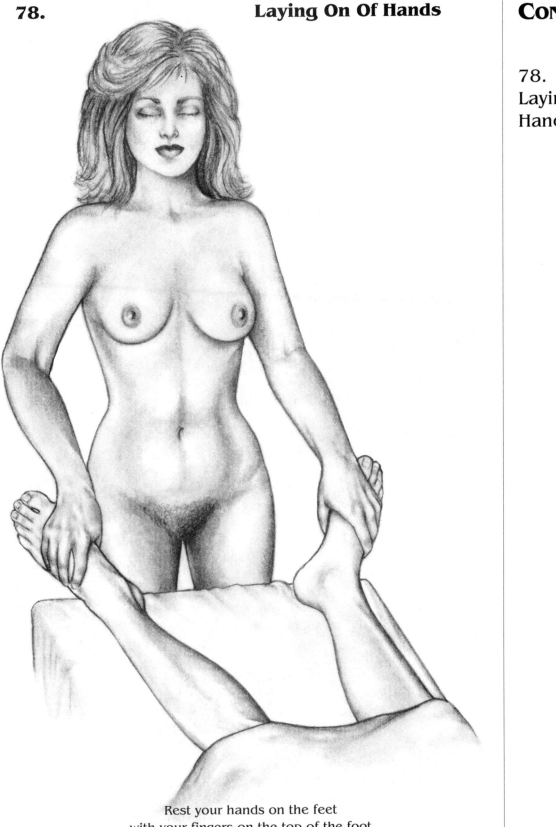

Rest your hands on the feet
with your fingers on the top of the foot
and the thumbs on the arches.
After a minute or so,
very slowly allow your hands to ascend off.

~

Remain quiet until your beloved returns to this world.

~

Embrace.

APPENDIX

Eroticizing Safer Sex

Massage in general
　　　is considered in AIDS safer sex guidelines
　　　to be a no-risk or very-low-risk activity.

When there is uncertainty
　　　about the giver's or receiver's health
　　　or if either partner is communicable
　　　with the AIDS virus,
　　　　　you may wish to read the following.

Current research indicates that
　　　when blood, ejaculate, or vaginal lubrications
　　　come in contact
　　　with a broken skin or membranous tissue surface,
　　　the transmission risk may increase.

Should you prefer to follow AIDS safer sex practices
　　　when massaging the male or female genital area,
　　　it is recommended
　　　to wear latex or vinyl examination gloves,
　　　which you can purchase at a pharmacy
　　　　　or surgical supply store.

(Concerning infectious skin conditions,
　　　such as herpes lesions or venereal warts,
　　　it is recommended to entirely forego contact
　　　with the communicable area
　　　　　or to consult a medical professional.)

When using a latex product,
　　　apply only a water-based lubricant
　　　　　since oil can deteriorate latex.
　　　If the water-based lubricant contains nonoxynol-9,
　　　which can destroy the AIDS virus on contact,
　　　the protection will be supplemented.
　　　Some people, though, are sensitive to nonoxynol-9.

An alternative or an addition to wearing gloves
        in a male genital massage
        is to place a condom on the penis.
Try a few drops of water-based lubricant
        in the tip of the condom before unrolling it.
Some of the strokes in this book, however,
        are best suited for gloves without a condom.

At first, these protective measures
        might appear as intrusions or hindrances.
After exploration, you may find,
        as many others have,
that latex and vinyl examination gloves
provide some uniquely smooth sensations,
that the water-based lubricant inside the condom
creates heretofore unexperienced pleasures.

Eroticizing safer sex means
        letting go of expectations
        and allowing the discovery of new worlds.
Giving the touch of love,
        as in the sensual massage offered in this book,
        can bring us all closer
        to these new worlds of pleasure.

Acknowledgments

Louise-Andrée Saulnier was the collaborator in the first edition of this book. It was through her love, support, and encouragement that I was to write and publish this first book to illustrate genital massage explicitly, a project no other publisher was willing to touch. I greatly appreciate her.

My principal meditation teachers, Tarthang Tulku and Billie Hobart, were a major influence on this book though they taught little about massage or sexuality.

The underlying massage style in *Erotic Massage* evolved in the early days of humanistic psychology. I wish to express my gratitude to Margaret Elke, whose work in massage and sensuality has influenced many, and to the pioneering teachers at Esalen Institute.

The students and faculty of The Institute for Advanced Study of Human Sexuality in San Francisco have continuously supported my teaching massage as a means to bring the sensual and intimate qualities into the sexual expression.

I am indebted to Clark Taylor, Ph.D., and David Lourea, Ed.D., of the Sexologists' Sexual Health Project in San Francisco for their support in eroticizing safer sex. I am equally thankful to Molly Hogan, R.N., Norma Wilcox, R.N., and Sharon Miller, M.S.

Finding an artist with both the sensitivity and the willingness to illustrate the subject matter of this book was a major undertaking. The sensual, spiritual eroticism of Kyle Spencer graces the pages of *Erotic Massage*. Her abilities and expressions inspire me.

My dear friend, Ellen Gunther, M.D., provided the photography on which the massage technique illustrations were based.

I greatly appreciate the support from so many others in so many ways: Chris McMahon, Chyrelle D. Chasen, Clara Kerns, Joseph Kramer, Lynn Craig, Mary Jane Harper, Nora LaCorte, Pam Johnson, Sandy Trupp, Saunya Tolson, Vicki Folz, Wendell Lipscomb, as well as others.

About the Authors & Artists

The Author

After leaving academia, Kenneth Ray Stubbs, Ph.D., moved to the San Francisco Bay Area. There he became a certified masseur in 1973 and studied a wide range of Western and Eastern approaches to health and sexuality.

Personally, massage became a meditation, more like the movement of T'ai Chi Ch'una than Tibetan Buddhist sitting meditation. Combining these experiences with a tantric approach to sexuality, he developed seminars for couples of all sexual orientations and training programs in Sensate Therapy for sex therapists.

He is the author of several books on sensuality, sexuality, and intimacy, which have sold more than 500,000 copies.

The Collaborator

Louise-Andrée Saulnier, M.H.S., is a clinical sexologist residing in Quebec City, Canada. For the last two years she was the host of her own daily television talk show featuring human sexuality. She continues to appear frequently on radio and TV and is a popular speaker for the medical profession and other groups.

The Illustrator

Kyle Spencer, illustrator of the black-and-white images, is a young artist residing in the San Francisco Bay Area. Her art appears also in *The Clitoral Kiss* as well as *Tantra: The Magazine* and *Ecstasy Journal*.

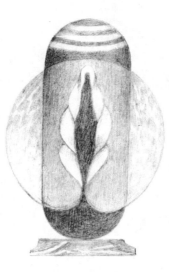

EPILOGUE

My beloved is gone down into his garden,
to the beds of spices,
to feed in the gardens,
and to gather lilies.

I am my beloved's,
and my beloved is mine:
he feedeth among the lilies.

The Song of Solomon 6: 2-3

This is the touch of love.